Dying To **BE THIN**

Advance Praise

"Dying to Be Thin is not a typical story of personal redemption. Ms. Gilbert writes from personal experience but offers practical solutions to those of us who have been suffering from the binge-purge cycle all our lives. While her story is completely different from mine as a man, her emotions and thoughts are exactly mine. The difference between *Dying to Be Thin* and therapy and self-help books is that her story gets inside your emotions to the reason you do this. She knows how you feel, and how to get out of that cave. I read it in an afternoon because I couldn't put it down. It's easy to read, but it's a book you'll come back to, making notes again and again."

– Brian Boyd

"Thank you to Noelle for sharing her story with us! I love how she gave us insight to her thoughts, upbringing, relationships, and how her bulimia affected her everyday life. I commend Noelle for everything she overcame and finding her strength to take control of her life. Even though I do not have personal experience with an eating disorder, the steps to overcoming bulimia were clear, simple to follow, and easy to maintain. The biggest part that I took from *Dying to Be Thin* is our mind and thoughts that we allow. If we allow ourselves to have a negative mindset, then it will become true. Noelle truly showed me that it is mind over matter."

– Dawnae Baldwin

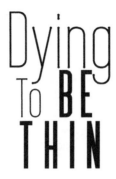

Dying To BE THIN

TOOLS *for* BATTLING *the* BULIMIA BEAST

NOELLE GILBERT

NEW YORK

LONDON • NASHVILLE • MELBOURNE • VANCOUVER

Dying To **BE THIN**
TOOLS *for* BATTLING *the* BULIMIA BEAST

© 2020 NOELLE GILBERT

Published in New York, New York, by Morgan James Publishing in partnership with Difference Press. Morgan James is a trademark of Morgan James, LLC. www.MorganJamesPublishing.com

ISBN 978-1-64279-724-4 paperback
ISBN 978-1-64279-725-1 eBook
ISBN 978-1-64279-726-8 audio
Library of Congress Control Number: 2019909850

Cover Design by:
Rachel Lopez
www.r2cdesign.com

Interior Design by:
Bonnie Bushman
The Whole Caboodle Graphic Design

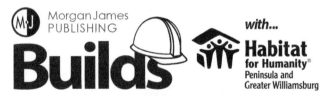

Morgan James is a proud partner of Habitat for Humanity Peninsula and Greater Williamsburg. Partners in building since 2006.

Get involved today! Visit
www.MorganJamesBuilds.com

To my three beautiful children:
Landon, Ava, and Brooklin.

Thank you for saving me.

TABLE OF CONTENTS

INTRODUCTION

I was standing with my back against the counter in the kitchen. Bobbie from the bank called, and there was an issue with my account. My funds were low, and once again the overdraft reserve had kicked in. Money was tighter than normal. My job was on the line; my work performance was declining substantially. It was getting harder and harder to finish my charting lately.

The binges had gotten so bad since the divorce that I was having a difficult time focusing on or even pretending to care about work. How could I have genuine compassion for others when my life was unraveling? Nursing was not my love. Not my passion. It was unfulfilling. Being the constant and stable figure for sick people who had no desire to help themselves out of their current predicament was exhausting. However, it was the few patients who I loved more than anything that kept me going. The bulimia was taking over. I would visit a patient in their home, rush through a fast-food drive through (or five), and then try to see another patient before the food settled. The fear of letting the food settle too long was always in the back of my mind. Haunting me. Causing insane anxiety and a sense of urgency to find a place to purge. If I waited too long, I couldn't throw up. I would hurry through another visit, do a pathetic job of assessing the patient, then speed to the nearest park or construction site that had a porta potty and try to vomit as much of the food as I could, only to have the desire to binge an hour later.

The cycle was vicious. Unforgiving. It continued over and over and over until my mind and body screamed for a break. My life was falling apart by the day. What if I couldn't pay my bills? What if I lost my job? I would lose my house. Would my ex take my kids away? Kids. Oh, my beautiful babies, they had been smack-dab in the middle of a ferocious storm through no fault of their own. Would they remember the crying, the yelling, the anger that I couldn't contain that was directed at myself but often overflowed onto their perfect little world? What if I couldn't take care of them?

Would I need to go to rehab? There's a place in California I have heard great things about. Some sort of holistic retreat. What if I made a huge mistake with my job? Would I lose my license? Five years and $35,000 wasted. What if the acid from my vomit continued to erode my esophagus? Destroy my teeth? The dentist had already made some curious comments about my enamel being thin and my gums looking overly inflamed. My esophagus couldn't continue the daily "vomit or no vomit" charade. My throat always ached. And there was a sharp pain under my right ribs. Was it my gallbladder? Stones, perhaps. Did I have an ulcer? It was usually when my head was in the depths of a fecal encrusted porta potty or behind a tree in some deserted area when these thoughts ravaged my mind.

I came back to the now. The bank. My account. Always something. I hung up and walked to the fridge. I opened it and stood there numbly. Did I really want to eat? I stopped for a moment before reaching in. Caught myself in the act—well, the pre-act. I thought to myself, "I'm not even hungry. Why am I wanting to eat? Sit down." My mind was pleading with me.

I shut the fridge and sat on the couch for a moment to try to decipher what I was feeling. Why the sudden urge to eat, to binge? It had been months since that urge had returned. What emotions was I feeling? How could I satisfy these emotions at this very moment without putting something in my mouth? I would not use food. I was going to let myself feel this time—the frustration, the disappointment, the anger, the annoyance. Don't use food. The thought played over and over in my mind until I started to get mad. Pissed. Enraged. I would not allow myself to be overcome by something that couldn't talk, couldn't feel, didn't breathe, couldn't reason or rationalize, didn't play any importance in my life but to give me blips of energy to sustain existence. I hated food. I thought that over and over. No other words at this moment could satisfy my absolute rage. I hated food! I wanted to scream. Wanted to reach across the counter and shake the bottle of coffee creamer. I wanted to throw the rice crispy treats from the cupboard that for years I so lovingly spread gobs of peanut butter on in the middle of the night. I wanted to rip the empty pizza box out of the garbage can and punch it until it was formless and limp.

Memories haunted me: the numerous times I drove to Jack in the Box to get a large Oreo cookie milkshake. That was usually the last stop on my thirty-thousand-calorie binges. It was thick and rich and disgusting in so many ways. Not to mention easy to barf up. I could recall the throw up burps that lasted for hours after I drank one of the creamy vanilla ones. Ugh. My stomach churned in disgust. I could recall the many times I threw the milkshake, half eaten, out the window of my car. I hated them. The smell, the taste, the look of the bright red maraschino cherry that appeared so deceptively perfect on top. "I hate food," was all I could think.

So why not? Why not go outside and throw the food against the house, the tree, the white vinyl fence? Why not let myself get angry at this object that haunted my waking dreams for years? This inanimate thing that destroyed my life. My health. My childhood. My marriage. My relationships. My career. Why not take a baseball bat, screwdriver, or sharpened pencil for all that mattered and drive it deep into the heart of the cream cheese–filled doughnut just to release the absolute hatred I carried around?

Because food is not the enemy. It's not the cause of this problem or the solution to any problem I have ever had. It isn't. Nor should it be. Why have I given food labels? Cursed it. Loved it. Had disgusting affairs with it and rendezvous at all hours of the day and night. At this point, I was standing back in the kitchen. Angry. Upset. Wanting to stuff my face with anything within reach. Oh, to feel numb. I walked upstairs and lay on my bed. Took a few deep breaths. "Let yourself feel," I chanted. I reminded myself of how amazing I was. How far I had come. I never imagined myself to be this strong. Never knew I had this kind of strength to overcome the demon that lived in the depths of me for so long. To conquer it. I had been pathetically weak for years. Given in to every temptation. How I looked forward to the moments of weakness because that was my out;

my pathetic excuse. My way to say screw it all and let myself have the sick desires of my heart: Costco cake, supreme pizza dipped in ranch, Cinnamon Toast Crunch with whole milk and maple syrup, mac and cheese with sliced fatty sausage stirred in it, fluffy croissants with butter and strawberry jam dipped in cream cheese frosting, anything and everything smothered in ranch, ranch, and more ranch.

But that depressed, overweight, weak girl had been dead for some time. She didn't even appeal to me. If anything, she turned me off to the point that even having her stop by for a few fleeting minutes repulsed me. She was no longer welcome. She could not cause me to relapse. As soon as she began calling, whispering sweet lies into my ears, filling my head with thoughts and ideas of momentary pleasure, she was shut down. Cut off. Oh, the empowerment from saying no was euphoric. Not a weak no, but a strong, empowering no. The act of saying no was more liberating than any binge I could ever imagine. I reminded myself that the feelings of momentary pleasure are fleeting. As the first few bites go down, it's bliss. The sweetness, the saltiness, the fat-laden richness of any morsel tasted heavenly for only a few seconds, but after that, it was torture. Sickening. During a binge I was mindlessly eating, and eating, and eating for, well, why was I eating?

I often forgot why. I wasn't hungry. Emotions. Yes, emotions. I didn't want to face them. That person is gone, but it took over twenty years of absolute misery and hitting rock bottom to realize just how much I wanted her gone. Since banishing her, my life has never been more amazing. My mind is clear. My body is lean and healthy. Punishing myself for fear of getting "fat" after a binge is a thing of the past. Every now and then I must remind myself of the person I was. A monster with an unquenchable demon inside. A monster that couldn't handle life. Couldn't deal with her emotions, unable to recognize how easy it was to feel and, in all honesty, too scared to let herself experience emotions.

A bulimic. Yes, a bulimic. For years all that consumed her was that undeniable desire to numb herself with food in hopes of shutting out anything that caused an unpleasant sensation inside her, followed by the need to purge from gorging on excess food and, when she really searched deep, knowing that she was killing herself. She was dying to feel, dying to love and forgive herself, and dying to be thin.

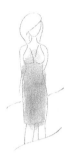

Chapter 1
LETTING GO OF
AN OLD FRIEND

A s you read this now, I want you to begin to sense your uniqueness. You are amazing in every way. Maybe you don't recognize it or believe it or see it, but I do. I write these words to reach a part of you that may have felt unreachable. Dead. Numb. Let my love and desire to help you resonate through you and flow into your life. You have passions, tastes, pleasures, fears, insecurities, and a personality that is unique. We share a common demon that must be eradicated so that you can be free to live a life of joy.

There is no "one size fits all" cure for any disease or disorder. I get a headache, I drink a Coke. You get a headache, you pop a Tylenol or two. Same problem solved by two different means. The same principle goes with treating your eating disorder. Yes, *yours*. Take ownership of it. In taking ownership, you deem that

1

it is yours to do whatever you wish with. In this moment, you are choosing to heal all of you and destroy the beast. No two people are identical in their needs with rehabilitation. I can vividly recall sitting uncomfortably in a cold leather chair in a therapist's office in Sacramento, California, trying to explain to him my feelings surrounding my bulimia. Why I hated myself. Why I used food as a means of self-inflicted torture and punishment. The contents of our conversations have blurred as the years have passed, but after seeing this therapist a few times, I realized our brief and cold encounters weren't making a dent in the problem. If anything, it was making it worse. Therapy may have helped, and continues to help others, but this form of treatment did not resonate with me.

You may have had the same issue. Conventional treatment is not working for you and the bulimia is worsening and intensifying daily. Your sense of urgency to fix your eating disorder is increasing to the point that battling the bulimia and finding a solution are all you can focus on. Your life is falling apart. You have hit a breaking point. Curing your eating disorder has become a mental obsession. Like I once did, you long to cure yourself, to stop being a slave to the relentless monster and start being a mom to your children and living a life you love and enjoy, free from the binge/purge cycle of bulimia.

For years, I dreamt of being able to spend a day with my children without binging or purging. I remember the nights where I would rush to feed my children dinner only to set them in front of the TV so I could stay in the kitchen and gorge myself into oblivion. I would finish the leftovers from dinner, then start on the unopened box of cereal in the cupboard, move on to my kids' school snacks and chips, and finish with a peanut-butter-and-jelly sandwich or two with a tall glass of whole milk. My son would peek around the corner and say, "Mom, you're still eating?" He didn't mean it hurtfully, but it was always a slap in the face that I was influencing them to have an unhealthy relationship with food. To eat themselves sick any time they felt unpleasant emotions. They were seeing erratic behaviors done in hiding. Their mom hoarding food. He could see the shame and embarrassment on my face after his innocent comment. Like I had been caught stealing or performing a heinous crime. Which I had. This is not what I wanted my sweet son to remember about his mother. I see a better world for you, as I did for myself not too long ago.

My dream for you is one I envisioned for myself years ago. Easy. Fun. Laughter. After an enjoyable meal with your family, I want you to sit around the table and play games. Watch a movie. Go for a walk or bike ride. Laugh at the park while you push your children on the swings. Make beautiful and needed memories with those sweet extensions of you that will one day be gone. I envision a world where you can sit down to meals with your children and family without the fear that you will lose control; a beautiful world where you no longer hide food or your eating, lie about eating, or steal food from your children's lunch boxes and then say you have no idea where the Twinkies and chips went; a world where you don't fear social gatherings where a vast spread lies before you; a world where the feeling of despair in your gut that purging is the only solution to a massive binge is gone forever; a world free from the anxiety and chaos that controls your day when you try to balance life with the binging and purging.

I want you to have a healthy relationship with food, a healthy relationship with yourself and the nonstop chatter going on in your mind. I want you to eat only what you need, to feel comfortable and satisfied, and to never feel stuffed or miserable. You deserve to have control and the power to say no to food and no to life's obligations that you cannot humanly fulfill. You deserve the power to change the thoughts that cause emotions and result in behaviors that keep the bulimic cycle alive and active.

I long for you to be in control of what is going on in your mind and life and therefore your mouth. This new world is magnificent. You appreciate food and enjoy its purpose. You use it to fuel you. I want you to wake up excited to live a glorious day and not be preoccupied, obsessed, depressed, or guilty for what you did or didn't do with your family: the unplanned vacations, the missed dates, staying home alone because you took a box of laxatives after a failed attempt to purge. Never again will you feel yourself missing out on amazing opportunities to be you and live life fully because of your bulimia. Your new world is calm and beautiful and optimistic in every way. Even when the world around you becomes out of control, you are mentally prepared and have the tools to overcome any obstacles. Your outside environment no longer contributes to your bulimia.

My ultimate desire is that you have absolute control over your bulimia so you can finally be an amazing parent to your children.

Problems with Conventional Treatment

From the outside, I looked like any other thirty-something single mom: decent-looking with an average body type, good job with security. Many would say I had it all together. My children were always well-groomed and well-behaved. I held down a busy nursing job and even found time to take my kids on day trips and outings around my small town every week. I drove a luxury car and lived in an expensive home. I was bright and happy when I entered the store, gym, or any local business in my town, and my presence brought a light that many couldn't help but be recognized. Everyone knew me. My smile and positive outlook were contagious. I had a strong desire to be honest and hardworking.

What the world didn't see was the loneliness, the sadness, the self-loathing, the negative and relentless chatter that went on in my head, or the crying in my bed night after night as I frantically searched the internet for "bulimia self-help groups," "bulimia treatment," "eating disorders and parenting," "emotional coping," "how to stop purging," and "eating disorders and sexual abuse." The world didn't see the bloodshot eyes, burst blood vessels, puffy face from water retention after a massive salt-laden binge, sore throat or hoarse voice from acidic stomach contents being brought back up, the rages of hate I threw for allowing myself to lose control with food and emotions, or the bloody knuckles that were repeatedly forced against my teeth in a desperate attempt to expel all the food.

I hid it all so well. Stress about having the money to support myself and my children permeates my thoughts. Questions like, "How I am going to handle another day at a job I don't like?" or "What if I lose my job because of my 'disorder,'" play like a broken record. It was getting more difficult to hold it together emotionally. I couldn't afford therapy/counseling any longer. How long had I been doing therapy now and still no results? Nothing helped. The therapist went over the same issues every week. We talked about the sexual abuse, the need to numb emotions, and the self-hatred. The feeling of being unloved and inadequate in every way made the problem bigger. It gave the problem more energy. I was done focusing on the problem; I wanted guidance to find solutions. No one understood how I felt. The therapist treated me like I was irrational and crazy. I longed to talk with someone who could relate to me, who understood. I needed help ending the binges, but the therapist didn't seem to offer any beneficial advice. He'd never been where I was. He'd never been face down in a filthy porta potty or corner gas station toilet. He'd never been so full of food that he couldn't walk, where any small movement made his abdominal skin feel as though it was going to rip open, allowing rotten food to pour out. He had never sat in front of another human and discussed why he absolutely loathed himself or cried night after night in desperation to find someone to relate to him.

I found it nearly impossible to locate an online treatment group that offered any helpful advice. "I just want to know that someone else understands me," I would think. "That would be more helpful than any treatment session." I knew I needed to work on handling my stress and my emotions, but no one seemed to be able to help. How do I go about changing my mindset—my outlook on life—anyhow? I felt lost. Alone. I couldn't continue down this path. My children were suffering the most. The time I spent battling bulimia was stealing precious moments I should be spending with my beautiful babies. They didn't deserve to be raised by a mom with bulimia. It had to end.

What if I did not fix this problem?

Bulimia is destroying my health? No freaking way! I say this with sarcasm, but the terrifying reality is that for a lot of years, I had no idea how much I was damaging my body. I was dumb and naive in so many ways.

Stomach acid is meant to destroy bacteria and digest food. You can only imagine how much bacteria passes through the stomach that must be destroyed and the very acidic environment of the stomach. Of course, there's a reason it's called *stomach* acid; it is meant to stay in the stomach. The stomach is composed in a certain way to make sure it can handle the toxic nature of its contents. When that acid comes barreling back up the esophagus and out of the mouth and body, the fragile and delicate tissues in the throat and mouth are exposed to it, not to mention the teeth, which are being destroyed slowly each time you vomit. Yes, destroyed. Vomit is destroying your esophagus, mouth, and teeth.

Every time you purge, you lose fluid and electrolytes that the body needs to function normally. Binges consist of thousands of calories of nonnutritive food that get vomited up again and again. The body is not getting the vital nutrients its needs. Sorry to disappoint you, but I can't recall in twenty years ever binging on apples, oranges, or kale! It's always "crap" food. Processed, color-filled garbage that leeches from the body to be broken down. Hair starts to fall out, become brittle, and appear unhealthy due to lack of nutrients. Skin starts to dry and crack. Nutrients are taken from bones and other vital organs. These are all signs that the body is lacking critical vitamins and minerals. These outward expressions are the body's way of screaming out in desperation, begging for help to stay alive and well. The loss of electrolytes and fluid can affect anything from the heart to the kidneys, resulting in cardiac arrest or kidney failure, not to mention the swelling from excess salt consumption and dehydration from vomiting.

Binges and purges are emotionally and physically exhausting. The out-of-control and consuming nature of the beast results in depression and anxiety. There is nothing positive about binging or purging. I can say without any hesitation that twenty years of my life was stolen from bulimia. My complete obsession with what I was going to eat, when, and where was all I could think about for many years. The fear of being discovered kept me in this dark cave of depression and anxiety for many of those years. I was terrified to eat in front of people for fear of being exposed or allowing anyone to see me out of control and my erratic eating behaviors. The anxiety felt from hiding the demon is not easy. It has only been the past two years or so that I am not ashamed to say I was a bulimic and am now fully recovered. No one wants to take a girl on a date and spend thirty dollars on her meal if he thinks she is going to run to the bathroom and vomit after.

Talk about having no social life. Feeling isolated because of your disorder is beyond depressing. If I was on a date and ate too much, I would want to rush home so I could continue to eat and eventually purge. Once the floodgates had been opened it was very difficult to stop the momentum, and I would continue in an ongoing binge. I often turned dates down or made excuses about having to leave afterward if I had taken a box of laxatives that day. It made me anxious. Paranoid. I was terrified of crapping my brains out in the presence of anyone, fearful and anxious about messing myself at work or school or while out running errands because of the uncontrollable bowel contractions that excess laxative use causes. The chains and bondage that the anxiety held me in was torture. I am amazed I was able to hold down a steady job and do a half decent job at being a mom because of the mental preoccupation bulimia caused. It's always there; it never sleeps. You wake up to it and go to bed with it. It is all-consuming and unforgiving.

Time stolen from my children is the one side effect of an eating disorder that trumps the others. My poor babies. My poor, sweet babies. Children are so sweet and loving, not to mention forgiving. I am truly ashamed to mention how many nights I left them alone to go binge and purge for hours on end. If I came home and they were awake, I would be furious and take my frustration out on them. I hated myself and what I was doing; therefore, it leaked into their lives. Not intentionally, of course. There would be mornings when they would come down to the kitchen for breakfast and find me on the floor crying out to God. They would be so confused and troubled, always asking, "Mommy, what's wrong? Are you sick?" How could I do such a horrible thing to them? All I ever wanted to do was love and shelter them from seeing me loath myself, but bulimia had taken over. The beast had devoured me. It consumed all of me. During the worst years of my bulimia, I was not able to be that fun, loving mom I always imagined was deep inside. Yes, I was amazing at times, but I cared more about and gave more attention to my addiction. To eating. To numbing. To having my head face down in the toilet retching. You cannot be a high-quality parent and have an eating disorder. You can't. It's not possible. Bulimia takes so much time. It is truly an all-consuming disorder. It permeates your mind when it's not ravishing your body. The obsession of it will destroy your life. Every aspect of it. I had to finally heal myself so that I could take the time and energy and focus it on being an amazing mom who was loving and patient with her children.

The amount of money I was spending on food was outrageous, yet I would complain when I had to pay for my children's sports or school activities. Talk about selfish! Add up all the money you are spending on binges and think of the things you could be paying off, paying for, or simply saving. Most binges would cost anywhere from forty to eighty dollars.

Just like a drug addict or alcoholic, I stopped caring about the cost; I simply wanted another hit. Once I stopped bingeing, I was able to pay off debt and bills quicker. It was amazing!

When it came down to it, I was afraid to give up my connection to food. Just like any addiction, it's not easy to give up a confidant. There was some sort of sick comfort that came from knowing if I had a rough day, I could go binge. A part of me wanted to eat all the wonderful and tasty deserts that others would deny themselves. I looked forward to going home at night after work and sitting down to an enormous plate of salty pasta with bread and butter. It brought a feeling of comfort. It was like walking into my home after being on a long vacation: the scent of vanilla, the softness of my couch, the enveloping feeling when I crawled into my own soft bed. It was reassuring and loving. Food didn't judge me, disagree with me, put up a fight, or make me feel not good enough. It was simply there. Observing. Ready to serve me whenever I needed it to. Food was my best friend for many years.

Or so I thought. I allowed it to take on a sick role in my life until I awoke to the realization that it wasn't my friend. It wasn't my confidant. It was destroying my life, not improving it. Like any friend, if it is not serving you in greater ways, uplifting you, making you strive to be better than you are at this moment, then it must be cut off. You don't need a friend who controls your life, who makes you hate yourself, who leaves you down in the depths of despair after the initial high of being with them. Think of the freedom you are gaining by leaving it behind. Stop telling yourself that you love food, that you can't live without it, that it's too hard. Those are comfortable lies that your mind replays over and over.

We will soon eradicate these lies from the hard drive of your mind. Do not underestimate your worth by allowing those lies to run your life any longer!

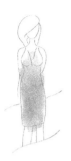

Chapter 2
MY BATTLE WITH
OVERCOMING THE BEAST

I was raised in a small town in Northern California. Amazing parents. Large family. Hot summer days in the pool and helping dad load cattle in the shute in the warm evenings. Picking cherries in the orchard and walking from house to house to sell them in the fall. Riding my bike to the corner gas station to buy atomic fireballs for five cents during the rainy winters. So many wonderful memories!

My childhood was much like any young girl's, except that, for reasons I did not remember at the time, I started overeating at a very young age: sneaking and hiding food, lying, stealing. All in the name of one more "hit" of a drug that I couldn't survive without. Sadly, we must eat to exist, so cutting out food is not an option.

One of my first memories was eating a tub of ice cream in my best friend's bathroom. I remember feeling horribly sick and wondering why I had done that to myself. I was about twelve years old. These binges became more frequent. Grade school came and went. The binges steadily grew in frequency. Middle school flew by. The binges were kept at bay because I began to put on weight, but when my emotions were intensified, so were the binges. Then came high school, a pivotal point in my life. In ninth grade, I began having bad dreams. They were vivid and disturbing. I wasn't sure why I was having them. During these high school years, my binges became worse than ever. I would eat a ridiculous amount of food, and even though it made me feel horribly sick, it brought about a wonderful feeling of numbness. If I ate enough food, stuffed myself to the point of sickness, I felt very few emotions. What an amazing discovery, or so I thought. It took away the feelings caused by the disturbing dreams.

One day after school, I ate myself into a complete stupor. I sat in the recliner next to the window that overlooked the valley and couldn't handle it any longer. No one was home. I had to release the intense pressure in my stomach. I walked into the bathroom off the kitchen, lifted the lid, and knelt on my knees. Was I really doing this? It felt foreign, not to mention disgusting. When had this toilet last been cleaned? It was a new experience in every way. I placed my left hand on the side of the toilet bowl and forced my right index finger down my throat. I vomited. Massive amounts of half-digested food came up with a force and small drops of toilet water splashed back up on my face. It was such a release, a euphoric feeling of power and control, but also sickening and physically exhausting.

I began throwing up a few times a week; then it became a daily occurrence. It took so much out of me physically that others could tell something wasn't right. I wasn't my usual overly energetic self. My mom was one of the first to notice. A few months after the purges began, she sat me down and asked what was going on. She had discovered vomit in the toilet and noticed my complexion was different: pale, sick-looking. I couldn't hide it any longer. I told her about my dreams and how real they felt. How disturbing they were. I was feeling so many emotions inside me and was not sure how to handle them. I confessed to her about my binges and how the purges started in hopes to relieve my aching stomach. I told her of how insanely euphoric it felt but that it made me feel horrible afterward. I hated myself for it.

She told me about the sexual abuse that occurred when I was a little girl. She wasn't sure how long it had taken place, but she and my dad had stopped it as soon as they found out and the offender was far away and unable to hurt me. She wasn't sure why the dreams were occurring now, so many years later. I must have blocked the memories out in an attempt to protect myself, but something recently triggered the memories. Emotions overcame me, flooded my body. At that moment, I hated the memories. I hated the offender. I hated myself. I blamed myself. I felt unlovable and unworthy. I was terrified to feel the emotions that were bottled up inside me.

Consequently, I continued to self-medicate with food. I ate. And ate. And ate. And threw up every chance I got, just to feel that euphoric release and keep myself from putting on more weight. I began a vicious cycle of binging and purging. The cycle was a release but also a form of torture, a way to punish myself. I must have been a bad and unlovable girl because someone had abused me. My parents encouraged therapy. I reluctantly went to a few therapy sessions, which were a complete waste. I took medication for a while, which seemed to help a little. The bulimic cycle only worsened. It continued through high school, college, and into my marriage. Hiding it was exhausting. It was almost more than I could handle, living so much of my life in secret, lie after lie.

In 2013, after my divorce, my bulimia spiraled out of control. My ten-year marriage had ended. I became a single mom of a one-year-old, two-year-old, and three-year-old. I was working full time and overwhelmed. Being twelve hours away from my family made me feel disgustingly alone and isolated. Alone and depressed, I turned to food for comfort. My best friend had returned. My companion. My confidant. It was always there to comfort me. I felt myself step back in time to my younger years and began to numb myself heavily with food. Even though I had had a handle on the bulimia for many years and kept it at bay during my marriage, the monster had reared its head when my life spiraled out of control, as it often does. I began binging and purging multiple times a day. It consumed me. Food was my drug of choice, not because I wanted it to be, but because it was available and convenient. It was comfort. It was what I knew. How lucky I am that I did not turn to drugs or alcohol. God was protecting me for sure. How merciful he is.

I hit rock bottom one night when I returned home to three crying babies who should have been sleeping. I had left them alone for a few hours to go have a massive binge after a completely horrific day at work. One of the kids had woken up and couldn't find me. The one child woke the other two children up and they were all terrified and crying when I returned. That night, the binge was bad. My abdomen ached. I looked six months pregnant. I cried all the way up the hill to my house for God to take me. It would be better to drive off the cliff and die than to continue like this.

Instead, I came home to three terrified children who needed a mom. Three beautiful babies who deserved a stable and constant figure who loved them and devoted her time to them and not her disease. After putting them back to bed, I went to my bathroom and tried to vomit. I gagged and dry heaved for over an hour, but nothing would come up. I had waited too long and the food had settled. That feeling of being so full of food that I could hardly walk was sickening. Like a balloon about to pop. The worst feeling anyone could imagine.

God had performed a double header that night. He had prevented me from vomiting so I could remember for hours afterward how horrible this feeling was. Also, he made it so my children's anguish was so raw and vivid that I couldn't unburn it out of my mind. I had to stop. Bulimia was consuming me. Destroying every part of my life. I looked in the bathroom mirror after the hour of desperately trying to vomit and cried. My eyes were bloodshot. I had burst a blood vessel in one of my eyes. I was hoarse and could hardly speak. My face was puffy and red. My knuckles had open sores on the tops from rubbing against my teeth for an hour. I was killing myself.

That's all I could think: "I am killing myself. My kids will grow up without a mom if I do not end this now."

It was that night that I promised myself that no matter what, I was going to heal myself. I didn't care what it took or how long it would take, my children would never again wake up to an empty home with an absent mother. They would never find me on the kitchen floor crying out in anguish to the Creator to remove the beast inside me. I would devote all the time I was wasting on my addiction and pour it into being a phenomenal mom and living a life helping others conquer their bulimia battle. My kids deserved a kind and loving mom and not a monster who hated herself and her life. It wasn't an overnight fix. It would take time. There might be relapses. It was small steps that I vowed to take every day, no matter how difficult, that would lead to monumental victory of overcoming this demon. I took ownership of my disease. I made it mine, and in doing so, I made it my choice to eliminate it. After twenty years of feeling like a helpless victim, a slave, a cowering puppet at the mercy of the master, I allowed myself to take complete power back. I was in control. I was taking back my life and the countless hours that bulimia had stolen from me and my children.

Let Me Guide You to the Light: My Vision of Freedom for You

Imagine that you're trapped in a dark cave, completely alone. It's cold, damp, and deathly silent. You aren't 100 percent sure how you got here, but now that you have opened your eyes to the reality of your situation, it's suffocating. You need to escape the darkness, to somehow get back to the outside world, to reality or what we call reality. You begin to stand up, but you can't. You're frozen. You try to move to the left. Nothing. Then you attempt a jerk to the right. Nada. The darkness is thick, but you recognize there is something holding you down, binding you. Heavy and cold. Chains? What on earth? How did you come to have these chains around you? All you want is to be to be free from the heaviness of the chains binding you.

There is no solution. No one to rescue you. No one within range to hear your screams. You mentally exhaust every option of freedom. Nothing makes sense. You give up, defeated. Hopeless. The fight is done, and you will end up dying here alone in a dark cave bound by some unseen object that keeps you frozen with fear. How did you get to this point? What led you down this road? Why does it all seem so overwhelming now? Could you have prevented this? What could you have changed? What if you had your life to live over again? Oh, how you wish to be free. You would do things differently. You plead to God pathetically.

After pleading for what seemed like hours, you feel the chains begin to loosen. Now you're able to shimmy a few inches to the left and right. Your lungs expand beneath the chains. You can breathe deeper. You begin to have hope. You know without a doubt that these restraints will soon come free, just be patient. Your mind reassures you. Believe. A new sense of hope and excitement begins to well up inside you. This is it. It would take time, maybe a few more hours, but the binding hold of these unbreakable restraints would eventually be loosened enough for you to break free. You no longer fear, no longer worry, no longer doubt. You notice a small light coming from behind what appears to be a large boulder at the far end of the cave. It's another sign, another empowering glimpse of what is coming. "My Creator, I believe. I will no longer take this life for granted. I will no longer hurt myself. I will release all these ungodly thoughts and false beliefs that have poisoned my mind. I will no longer abuse myself. Punish myself. I have been waiting for so long to be free, and now I see the light. It's there. There is hope!"

By the time the chains are loose enough for you to slip them off, you are exhausted mentally and physically. You have been fighting for what feels like an eternity. You push your weak body up and walk toward the small guiding light in the corner of the cave. It becomes larger and larger until it opens into a small entryway. You squeeze your body through a narrow space and out into the sunlight. You step out onto the sand. Your feet are bare, and you can feel every sensation against your skin. The sand encloses your feet as you walk across it. The sun brings an overpowering feeling of warmth. It's amazing. It feels like freedom. Like hope. The bondage is gone. You have a new passion. A new reality of what your new life will be like. All you had to do was believe you could break the chains.

I want you to take my hand for a moment. I want you to give me your undivided trust. I want to take you on an amazing journey. It won't be easy. At times it won't be fun or exciting. You may want to pack your bags and go back to the comfort of who you were. Back to the comfort of your habits and your ways of existing. Even if they aren't the best ways, and possibly even destructive, it's what you know. Those destructive ways have not served you up to this point, so I plead that you will let them go. God has placed a desire in my heart to guide you, to reach out and lead you down this amazing path that I traveled not too long ago. Although the path may seem dark and hopeless right now, if you allow me to, I will help you find that small light in the darkness that leads to freedom.

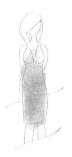

Chapter 3

WHAT'S TO COME — HOW AM I GOING TO BATTLE THE BEAST?

My amazing friend, come along with me as we embark on an exciting adventure of healing. Search deep within you and find that strength that we both know is there and turn that doubt to belief. Overcoming the bulimia beast has never been easier. Decide now that you will conquer this fight once and for all. You can. You will. With your hand in mine, I will guide you down the path of freedom. Below is a brief overview of what is to come in the following chapters:

In chapter 4 you will uncover your *why*, the reasons for wanting to overcome your eating disorder. With the help of the impact scale, you will understand the importance of your *why*; your reasons for overcoming bulimia long term and understanding how your *why* will play a critical role in preventing future relapses.

I will provide you with the tools and knowledge to stop the most damaging and destructive part of the binge/purge bulimic cycle in chapter 5.

Chapter 6 will divulge the valuable tools to break the second-most-destructive part of binge/purge cycle: the binges. Binges start the cycle and are followed by the purging, and play into the compelling need to vomit.

Together in chapter 7 we will uncover your emotions and help you to realize how your feelings factor into the bulimic cycle. You will discover methods to help change your thinking and prevent the behaviors that follow.

Chapter 8 will assist you in recognizing how a higher power factors into overcoming your bulimia. You are never alone in this fight for freedom.

At the end of chapter 9, you will know that you no longer have to punish yourself with other compulsive behaviors such as laxative abuse or obsessive exercising. These behaviors can be just as damaging as the binges and purges.

At the end of chapter 10, you will be able to identify solutions to help you prevent and overcome future relapses.

Free at last. Yes, free! Chapter 11 will show you how you can have long-lasting freedom. You will understand how you can heal yourself from bulimia; though it might be challenging, you can overcome these obstacles easier and quicker if you put trust in me and do the process with me guiding you along the way.

My dear reader, I am just like you in many ways. I am a mom, a friend, a lover, a daughter, a sister, a nurse, an employee, a solver of problems, a handyman, a cook, a maid, a warm-blooded, child-rearing ball of energy and cells with a deep sense of spirituality and love. I *was* also a fearful food-driven binger, self-loathing purger, emotionally numb and obsessed lover of delectable morsels. I was a hater and lover of rich, creamy, sugar-laden fried comfort food, a craver of heavy, toxic sustenance to stop me from feeling, a practicer of this Jekyll-and-Hyde eating disorder. No one saw this hideous side of me. I hid it for years.

Is this you? Do you feel as though you are living a Jekyll-and-Hyde life right now? Is the beast inside you on the verge of rearing its head? Have comfort. The days of looking six months pregnant after a binge are almost gone. The unstoppable robotic hand-to-mouth action that won't cease is at its end. The overpowering need to consume any food in sight is being phased out. Feeling bound and captive by the addictive power of food is no longer. We cannot escape food. It is all around us. We must eat to live out an amazing life. Our bodies need nutrients; there is no denying that. But gone are the days that you live to eat, and eat, and eat. I was all those things listed earlier until I found that I no longer had to be. You, too, will realize that freedom is near. You can have a normal and healthy relationship with food and with yourself that will free up time and energy that you never imagined. Just as I slayed the bulimia beast once and for all, you too can destroy the monster that's been skulking beneath the surface.

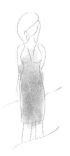

No human wants to live with an addiction. No human wants to be controlled by an outside object. We all wish to be free and peaceful with our thoughts and actions. Being a slave to your thoughts, to food, to destructive habits and behaviors, is not living. It's dying. Start living my friend. Start waking up every day and thanking God for the opportunity to go about this glorious day in complete freedom. Why do you want to overcome bulimia? Why do you want to prevent future relapses? Why do you want to free up time and energy to devote to your family and your children or enjoying life's experiences? I sit here and ponder on what your "why" might be, and I become exhilarated. Your why for doing anything in life ignites that fire deep inside you. Excitement. Passion. The insanely happy and giddy feeling that overcomes you to know that you can accomplish anything. The driving force for your cause. Maybe your why is subtle. Maybe it was a monumental event that opened your eyes. Whatever it is/was, it stirs up inside you a reason for beating this beast. For taking back your power. For gaining control and living life to the fullest. Once you have slayed the monster, you can conquer all things. Absolutely nothing can hold you back. Let's discover what your *why* is!

Impact Scale

I want you to take out a notebook or notecards and list all the things that are currently being impacted by your bulimia. If I were to have done this a few years ago, it would have looked something like this:

Kids. Job. Social life. Health. Weight. Happiness. Sense of freedom. Enjoyment with life in general. Finances. Connection with a higher power. Mental state (increased anxiety and depression).

Your list is going to look very different than mine, and it may be longer or shorter, but that is more than fine! Next, I want you to list your impact scale points in order of what/who is most impacted by your bulimia. What is being destroyed or suffering the greatest? Mine would have looked like this:

Kids. Happiness. Mental state. Enjoyment in life. Job. Social life. Weight. Sense of freedom. Connection with a higher power. Finances. Health.

As you can see, there are some points that are similar (such as happiness and enjoyment in life), and that's just fine. Points that others would consider critical, like finances, are toward the bottom of my list. Everyone's order of importance will vary. At my lowest point with battling bulimia, some things did not feel as urgent as others. Finances and my health took a back seat. They were critical, but my children, happiness, and mental state were a priority.

Next, I want you to take the top three on your list and write them on three separate pieces of paper or note cards, whatever is easiest. My children were number one on the impact scale, hands down. My happiness with life and who I was came second. How my mental state was being impacted came third. I wrote these on three separate note cards and left the back blank for the next step.

If your bulimia goes untreated, how will your life be impacted in each of these areas? How will your health, job, kids, and finances be affected? I want you to write down as many reasons as you can think of. My reasons for each point are listed below:

Kids

They are being neglected in every way. I am not spending quality time or enjoying life with them. They are seeing outbursts of anger/rage. Observing a mom who hates herself. Watching me use food to numb or cope and having an unhealthy relationship with food. I am setting my children up to have that same horrible relationship with food. I am killing myself and my children will grow up without a mom if I don't stop.

Happiness

I am unable to enjoy life when there is a constant preoccupation with eating and barfing. I can't be happy when I am controlled by something else, mentally and physically. I am unhappy because of the time and money I am spending on my disease, not to mention the destruction of my health. Others are suffering with this disease, and I long to transform others' lives. That would bring me complete happiness. It makes me to sick inside to think of others going through this alone, that they are living in unhappiness just as I am. I feel so alone, living with this secret; hiding this monster inside me steals and my happiness I have. I can't be truly happy living with bulimia.

Mental State

I feel as if I am crazy. My mind races constantly, obsessed with all the food that sounds good that I am dying to binge on to numb myself. What am I going to eat? Where am I going to eat it at? How much? I need to be cautious not to eat too much, or certain foods, or it might not come back up. What things are easiest to vomit? Where should I go to purge? Then there is the mental embarrassment of ordering so much food. Where should I put the trash or wrappers from the binges? There are obligations I have that I need to work around. How much time do I have to eat and binge? I must give myself a few hours because of the way I look after I vomit. Do I have a few hours? Do I smell like throw up? Have I brushed my teeth after my binge? I need to drink water, so I don't dehydrate myself. Do I have gum to ward off throw-up burps? Should I take laxatives if I can't throw it all up? How long do I have before I start pooping? There is also the mental preoccupation with unfulfillment—I hate my job and where I am at in life—which leads me to eat to numb my emotions, feelings of insecurity and inadequacy. I am killing myself. The mental game is endless and absolutely exhausting.

I want you to read through the paragraphs you've written a few times at least. Read each of the reason statements slowly and feel each word as it passes in your mind or out of your lips. I want you to feel, yes, *feel* throughout your entire body, the emotions behind each statement. I began to cry as I read the words, "They are being neglected in every way" and "I am killing myself, my children will grow up without a mom if I don't stop" and "Others are suffering from this disease, I long to transform others' lives." They were the three statements that made me ache inside to read. They were the most real and harsh.

These three statements satisfied the question of why I am overcoming this fight. They were the most exciting to read. They gave me a sense of excitement and passion. Hope. They were my *why* for slaying the demon. The statements that you choose are your *why* statements and are the reasons you are fighting, overcoming, conquering, and leaving this bulimia monster behind! Write them on multiple notecards and keep them anywhere and everywhere you can, to be reminded *often* of your magnificent journey. You might need them when things get rough and you have a strong desire to give up and relapse. I am so proud of you. This can be an exhausting task emotionally. But you did it. You are beyond amazing. I love your strength!

My *why* has been there when I have wanted so desperately to give in. When I have been weak and unemotional to the exhausting battle I was waging. Yes, I had times when I wanted to stop caring and did not want to stop binging, purging, thinking destructive thoughts, punishing myself, or numbing with food. It is when you overcome and continue to push forward in those times of weakness that you realize your strength. Remember, you are not the only one involved in this war. You are fighting this fight for others as well. I had to remind myself this battle was for my sweet children, my mental stability and happiness, and those all around me suffering. I had to climb this mountain for them. I didn't want to be consumed with thoughts like those listed above any longer. I wanted a mind filled with beautiful and happy thoughts. With love and enjoyment. With peace, forgiving, and acceptance of myself and my life.

If you have been telling yourself that you are unable to conquer your eating disorder and food addiction, stop now! If you feel as though you will never truly enjoy life because of the obsession and compulsion to act on the bulimia, eradicate those lies right now. Do not let those false thoughts enter your mind again. I am here to tell you that you can and will overcome this. You can do anything. This demon inside you will be gone! You just have to believe. *Believe.*

——— CRITICAL POINT: ———

If you haven't already, write down a list of everything that is being impacted by your eating disorder. After you've listed them, decide which three are the most effected. List each item separately on a notecard. On the back of each of the three notecards write all the reasons that item is being impacted. Read each of your reasons and take the one that touches you strongly, and that, my friend, is your why statement! You will have three why statements that will ignite a fire inside you to overcome your bulimia.

You have your *why* statements that have lit a fire and began a stirring of excitement inside you; now let's delve into banishing the purges.

Chapter 5

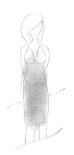

PURGE FREE—ENDING THE MOST DESTRUCTIVE PART OF THE BINGE/PURGE BULIMIC CYCLE

When people think of bulimia, they don't dwell on the binges or the emotional/mental issues that are behind the outward occurrences. They tend to focus on the purges: the vomiting, hovering over the toilet bowl with a finger down the throat and dispelling the food from a massive binge. Purging is by far the most physically destructive and damaging part of the cycle. When I say cycle, I am referring to the two main parts of bulimia: first, the binges or overeating to the point of discomfort, guilt, and other negative feelings; second, the purges, or the vomiting of stomach contents before complete digestion. The purging always follows a binge. Purging stomach contents is so damaging that it must be addressed first before any other part of the bulimia. Below are techniques that I used for years, and still occasionally use, to help me become (and stay) purge free. I beg of you to use them frequently and consistently (daily would be ideal) to receive the most benefits for eradicating the beast.

Jar O' Barf

Weird name, I know. Yet this is one of the most disgustingly useful techniques I have come across in deterring the desire to binge and/or purge. It works for both parts of the cycle. I remember when the purging became out of control after my divorce. One day while my head was hovering over the toilet bowl, I looked down and realized the absolute disgustingness of what I was looking at. Vomit: the smell, the taste, the look, even the sound of it as it was forcefully expelled out of my stomach and up my throat made my skin crawl. The chunks of partially chewed corn and lettuce from a pork salad. The little round brown balls from Reese's Puffs cereal. The thick white milky vanilla shake. Ugh. Vomit is so nasty! And even now, as a nurse, the one thing I cannot be within a few feet of, is vomit. Poop, sure. Blood and guts, no problem. Sweat, please—that's cake. Chewed up food in a slimy soup of bile and gastric juices, heavens no. It makes me ill even thinking about it now.

As I was saying, while my head was staring at this disgusting mess of what I binged on, I had an amazing idea. I had already slowed down on the frequency of the purges, twice a day was an improvement, but was having a heck of a time stopping them altogether or making them more infrequent. The idea of Jar O' Barf was an amazing concept to me. The thought occurred clearly: I should spoon some of this nasty mess in to a mason jar and every time I had the desire to binge/purge, I would open that jar that I kept concealed in the fridge and take a big ol' whiff!

Needed: Air tight jar, preferably glass, and as much or as little vomit as you wish.

Process: Place the jar in your fridge in clear sight and every time you have a desire to binge or purge pull the jar out, open it, and take a few deep breaths of the disgusting contents.

The first time I used this technique it was a little rough. I almost didn't do it because the thought alone made me want to vomit! The point of having a jar of throw up in plain sight sitting in your fridge is so that you can use it! Don't set it on the shelf and let it rot away while you continue to binge and purge. This technique is powerful. I had no desire to eat for a few hours. The smell was burned into my memory. I had to get fresh vomit from time to time, but purges became more infrequent as I performed this technique.

Maggot Visualization

This technique doesn't exactly have to be maggots. It can be any nasty creature or bug that makes your stomach churn and leaves you sick inside. I remember having an anatomy and physiology lab in college where we worked on cadavers. I recall seeing a small white bug looking thing writhing and thrashing around one day inside the rotten abdominal cavity of the cadaver. Lo and behold, it was a maggot. From that day, my disgust for maggots was out of this world. I was at home one evening making dinner for my children. It had been a rough day. The kiddos were being out of control. I was overwhelmed. The desire to eat started to creep up on me, became stronger and stronger until I wanted to eat and binge myself into numbness.

I opened the cupboard and grabbed the jar of peanut butter, my trusty go-to for starting a binge. For some strange reason, there was a small piece of stale bread in the bottom of the jar. At that moment the thought of a white maggot entered my mind and I became sickened. I screwed the lid back on and set the jar in the cupboard. I was disgusted. No way would I eat that now. It worked! From then on, every time I would think of peanut butter I would think of maggots. I also started doing this with cereal and milk, cottage cheese, certain fatty meats, and anything that appeared "nasty, fatty, soupy, or thick" like there could be a white maggot squirming around in it. I've gone so far as to tape pictures of maggots on the outside of containers to give me a beautifully wretched visual of what might be lurking inside. Works wonders! Talk about negative conditioning!

Needed: disgustingly vivid pictures of things that make your stomach churn (maggots, any nasty bug, snake, spider, even pictures of blood and guts if that makes you sick to your stomach).

Process: Pictures can be placed on food bags or containers to deter you from eating them.

Video the Reality of It—Literally

"I am killing myself. Killing myself." That was all I could think as I watched the video on my phone after one of my severe bulimia benders.

This was by far the hardest of the purge-free techniques that I have used. I remember looking in the mirror one day after a massive bender and thinking, man I wish I could see myself how I am right now *before* I start binging or purging. Then the idea came to me, I should video myself after binging and then again after purging and watch it every day. I got out my phone and recorded my next binge and purge. I began watching this video every morning after I did my "new self" meditation to reopen the wound just a little. Some days it reopened the wound a lot and left it gaping. I did this purge-free technique for only a few months because I did not like seeing myself in such a complete and utter state of agony. Watching the desperation and the pathetic visual of what I was doing was evident in my face and in my voice: the puffy, swollen cheeks stained with tears, the hate and sadness in my eyes and in my voice as I spoke hoarsely, bloodshot eyes, small blood vessels in and around the outside of my eyes bursting from the horrific force of vomiting. A few times I had bitten my lip while purging and blood had settled in the corners of my mouth. The video captured this vividly. It was an unpleasant sight. Talking on the video was beneficial for me.

I spoke a few sentences in a weak and defeated voice. Questioned why I was continuing this. Pleaded to myself that I didn't want to do this to myself any longer. Looked straight into the camera and said, "Noelle, you are killing yourself. You are destroying your life and your children's lives. This is not how you were meant to live."

The video was a vivid and depressing sight. It was truly a plea for help in moments of complete desperation. After a few months I stopped watching the video. I wanted to see myself in this low state, so I could be impacted, but I didn't like the negative nature of the video. The undesirable energy that resonated from it. That was not the person I wanted to be any longer. I wanted to see the new me, the best version of myself. After a few months I started focusing on my future "bulimia-free" self and not the reality of where I was currently. If we focus too much on the now when solving an issue, we often get more of it. My focus on the future became greater and more powerful. Every so often for the next year, after being completely healed, I would watch this video. It was a harsh reality of what I had done to myself for *way* too long. It was as thought I was watching a video of another person, but instead I was the main actor. I reminded myself (and still remind myself) of how the ending played out: the death of that actor. She was gone, no longer existed, was no longer welcome. In her place was a new and amazing actress who blew the old one out of the water. She resonated health, strength, power, confidence, self-control, beauty, and, above all, a love and zest for life.

Even years later, I remind myself that I am way too good to have an eating disorder. Yep, I am a borderline superhuman! So are you! Use these three powerful purge-free techniques to help you end the vomiting. Use them to help you recognize the disgusting reality that you are currently living in and that you *can and will* get past it. This is not where you are going to stay any longer. You no longer have to live like this. Stop killing yourself. Stop hurting yourself. Take out your *why* cards and tape them to your bathroom mirror. Put them in your car. On your kitchen cabinets. In the fridge. Anywhere you possibly can. Your *why* is greater than bulimia. Greater than the purges. Greater than the binges. Greater than those absurd negative thoughts swarming around in your head. My amazing children, my mental state, my happiness, and you, my dear friend, are my driving force. The light and power under my wings to set me soaring to health and happiness. You have the purge-free tools, now put them into action.

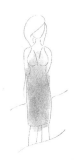

Chapter 6
BINGE FREE OR BUST

I
t was Thanksgiving 2014. I was at my good friend's house. I can remember it like it was yesterday. We had had a lovely Thanksgiving meal. I ate, but not in excess. I felt good about my ability to remain in control throughout the night as we cleaned up dinner and then corralled the children and put them to bed. As soon as the house was quiet, I went downstairs to the guest room. I had felt unusually stressed that day and the entire week, overwhelmed by kids, single parenting, life. Negative thoughts about myself and who I was started creeping in: insecurity, inadequacy, stress from my job. I had so many deadlines, charting, more and more training every week, Medicare changes. Rules. Rules. Rules. Healthcare was exhausting. An inner unease that had been there all day was growing by the second. I could feel the urge, the feeling

I always experienced when a binge was coming on, when the desire to numb the challenges of life began. After fifteen-plus years of living with this dark secret, I had learned to recognize all the signs, mainly the feelings and thoughts that surrounded the urges.

However, I never understood if this was more mental or physical in nature. Was it just a habit now? Had I let it become engrained in my daily routine? The thought of facing the demon mortified me; it sent a feeling of doom throughout my being. I waited a half hour. I knew my friend and her husband were upstairs in bed with their door shut. Sweat began to bead on my forehead and between my breasts under my sports bra. I hated binging at someone else's house, especially a close friend's. It made me nervous. I felt like a criminal performing a heinous crime and praying to a disappointed God not to get caught. Maybe I should go to the grocery store down the road or find a gas station. Anywhere else would be better. What would I tell her when she heard the front door open and shut? "Um, I snuck out at 11:30 at night to go binge on food. Yep, and all we've done today is eat!" Hmm. That would not make sense to anyone but a food-addicted, emotional-numbing bulimic. As someone who had always been thin, with impeccable self-control, and who had fought with me absolutely tooth and nail that food addiction wasn't real, my friend had no clue about the depth of my sickness.

I crept up the stairs and quietly opened the pantry door. Lord have mercy, the chocolate layer cake from dinner was sitting quietly on the shelf, beckoning me to indulge myself. Just one bite. It wouldn't hurt anything. But the one bite turned into two, then three, then six. It tasted heavenly. The release of endorphins was flooding my body once gain. The momentary pleasure was euphoric, but the voice in my head was screaming at me to stop.

Next thing I knew, I had devoured every ounce of the cake but a small sliver. Not even enough for one person. Well, enough for a person who practiced self-control. What have I done? My mind was racing. Guilt and shame overcame me. Self-loathing engulfed my being. Should I go buy another cake? Maybe I should eat all of it and make up a lie about what happened to it? Or play dumb. This had happened so many times before, you think I would have learned my lesson. I have made and remade more cakes, cookies, pies, PB&Js, and treats than I dare to admit. I slowly covered the pathetic-looking leftover chocolate cake and closed the pantry. I crept back downstairs and began to cry. Why? Had I really let myself become this person? Used food to numb out my emotions? Everything had been so hard since the divorce. So many years of living with this eating disorder. When was it going to stop? I hated myself. I loathed my existence. I hated what I did. I hated the lies and deceit and absolute lack of self-control. I despised food. My friend was going to be furious.

Livid. Of all times to have a binge. At least it wasn't two cakes. Or a gallon of ice-cream. I couldn't help but imagine maggots squirming in it. At this moment the thought of maggot-infested ice cream made me nauseous. On the plus side, there was no purging this time. No laxative use. No excessive exercising. No starving myself for days after. I could chalk it up to a small victory. I can't remember falling asleep. After what seemed like an hour of crying, the exhaustion overcame me. The sad reality was, it wouldn't be my last binge.

Imagine for a moment that you're a man who's just come home from a stressful day at the office. Your boss was a complete jerk today. No surprise. He reminded you a dozen times that the deadline for your notes on a project was getting close and your job was on the line if you didn't get them turned in on time. The pile of unfinished work on your desk was growing and the amount of extra time to complete it was diminishing by the day. You leave the office and drive home in silence. As you enter the front door of your home, the kids run up and begin an endless chatter of their school experiences. They pull your hand excitedly over to the table to show you what they've created and continue to give you moment-by-moment playbacks. Your wife hands you a to-do list then starts complaining about her day and how hard it is to be a stay-at-home mom. How exhausted she is, how stressed she feels. How the house isn't big enough for all of them any longer. They need more space. They can't afford to add on unless he gets a bonus. What should they do? Her tone becomes angry, frustrated. The thought of your boss staring down at you as you sit at your desk pops into your mind. A pit enters your stomach. You feel a boiling feeling welling up inside you. Pressure. Anxiety. Frustration. Annoyance. You yell, "Stop! Give me a second to relax. Dad needs a timeout." You walk downstairs and sit on the couch in the dark. Quiet. Calm. "My mind needs a rest," you hear yourself say out loud. The boiling feeling begins to subside, you start to feel a handle on all the ropes that are pulling you every which way. After giving yourself fifteen minutes of peace, you walk back upstairs and are ready to be a dad and husband. Ready to be present. You were able to handle the stress of life with ease.

Binging is the second most destructive part of the binge/purge cycle. The first story was a personal reflection of one of my many binges. People who suffer from bulimia do not handle emotions in a healthy or productive way. If they did, there would be no reason to gorge themselves. No reason to numb. No reason to use food as a self-induced punishment or a means of emotional release. The second account is how people *should* handle a stressful situation. They assess it and recognize they have emotions that they need to address. They release emotions in a healthy way. Most importantly, they take the emotion in, feel it, acknowledge it; then they let the emotion go, allow it to dissipate from their mind and body, and recognize it does not need to be destructive by holding it inside or continuing to mull it over. It's gone. Easy.

"Great, Noelle," you're saying, "but how do I stop binging?" Well, you must understand that a huge driving force to binge is having inner turmoil. Negative or destructive thoughts that turn into negative and destructive emotions, leading to a build-up of energy inside us that needs be released. Ideally, in a healthy manner. Below are the "binge-free techniques" I used for years to get myself to lessen the binges and eventually end them altogether. I use many of them still and know that my positive and healthy relationship with food is because I took the time to perform these techniques for many years. As silly, mundane, or simple as they might appear, it's the act of repetition that saved me. And it will save you.

Don't Tempt the Weak; Remove Obstacles

I know you have heard this over and over, but, boy, is it legit! Don't buy food that tempts you! For years I would not buy regular butter, peanut butter, certain white breads, most baked goods, sugary cereals, ice cream (still do not), and syrup. These were my go-to foods. Once I started to eat any of them, it was a downward spiral of sugar cravings, salt cravings, and fat cravings, repeated over and over. I would put peanut butter in my sugary cereal and pour syrup on top. I would take a heaping spoonful of peanut butter and mix it in a tub of ice cream and warm it in the microwave for a few seconds until it was soft and stirred in nicely. I would put gobs of salty butter on all baked goods and then dip them in syrup. Yep, I had an issue. An addiction. Once I stopped buying "binge foods," it became harder to eat as much as I needed to numb myself. I ran out of things to eat. I would let my kitchen become bare on purpose. I still occasionally do. More out of laziness now, not for fear of binging. When I was healing myself from bulimia, I refused to buy food for my children that I knew would be a temptation for me, no matter how bad they wanted them! I still refuse to buy certain items just as a precaution. I only buy school snacks that I know I will not be tempted by. I will not put myself in harm's way by buying yummy items that call my name in the middle of the night. That stare deep into my soul when I open the cupboard of fridge. I am extra cautious and protective of where, what, and how I order things at restaurants. It takes only a moment of weakness to fall back into old habits and allow a very subtle beast to reenter the picture. Even though I know I would never purge again, I am cautious about not allowing myself to open the floodgates to a binge. Period!

Another way to remove obstacles is being aware of how you respond to certain situations. If you know that you become stressed in the morning, or when the kids get home from school, and get the urge to binge, then change it. Change up your routine. Do ten minutes of yoga or sit and have a cup of tea before the kids rush through the door. You must change the situation or change your response to it, or both. Go to the gym in the morning to make yourself feel good and release some stress first thing before work. I absolutely love the definition of insanity: repeating the same thing over and over expecting different results. I can't say it any better. If you know a situation in your life causes a definite outcome, slowly work on changing it.

Before you eat a meal, ask yourself how hungry you are. Some days, I will eat only within a four- or five-hour window during the day. Intermittent fasting allows me to be more receptive and in tune with my inner self, especially when the body does not have the extensive burden of breaking down and digesting food. When I eat, I become full very quickly. I love the feeling of true hunger. It makes eating so satisfying and beautiful. However, we must be cautious of our emotions and how sneaky they can be! I will have a desire to eat when I am feeling emotional, and I make sure to question if this is true hunger or not. Weather you eat six meals a day or one meal a day, ask yourself before you eat if you are truly hungry and take a second to become aware of what emotions you are feeling. Emotions cause us to eat. Smells cause us to eat. Social situations and pressure cause us to eat. Those are not causes of true hunger. They are things that trick the brain into thinking it wants to eat, but it does not.

——— **CRITICAL POINTS:** ———

- A huge driving force to binge is inner turmoil: negative or destructive thoughts that turn into negative and destructive emotions, leading to a build-up of energy inside us that needs be released and manifests as actions.
- Do not buy food you know you will eat in excess. Period.
- Do not buy "comfort foods" that you have an emotional connection to.
- Go out for treats. Make it fun and special. Enjoy it!
- Before eating or throughout the day, ask yourself how you are feeling. Are you eating your emotions or are you eating because you feel true hunger?

Pre-Meal Mantra to Relax the Body and Calm the Mind

One characteristic of many (not all) bulimics is impulsivity. I know for sure this is spot on about me. When a binge would begin, I took on a "I don't give a rip and screw it all" attitude. No bueno! Instead of prioritizing meals and sitting down (don't raise your hand if you stand up when eating), we quickly rush through mealtimes and gobble food up in a matter of minutes when it takes the body twenty to thirty minutes to register "I am full so slow down." One technique I have taken on is the act of saying a premeal mantra in my head before I eat or drink. Every now and then I forget to do this, but I strive to say my mantra before meals because it helps calm and relax me while eating. I love the feeling of control and awareness it showers over my body. If I am out with friends or family or around someone who does not know I do this, I will usually take a few deep breaths then recite my mantra in my head before I take my first bite. I keep my mantra to myself because many would consider it odd. However, the concept of intuitive eating has become more popular over the past few years and is a phenomenal way to begin any meal. Feel free to tweak this mantra or create your own amazing one, long or short, but these are the words I say:

"I am grateful for this food (or drink) I am allowing inside me and how it nourishes my body. This food floods me with light and energy. This food helps me live a life of happiness and enjoyment. Right now, I am calm. I am at peace. I am in full control. I have no need to rush eating because there is an endless abundance of food. I am always in control. I love myself. I love food. I love our peaceful interaction."

My mantra is longer than some would like. However, it includes the most important aspects I want to emphasize between myself and food and how we interact. It reminds me that there is an abundance of food and no need to feel scarcity.

My premeal mantra gives me time to calm down and not start mindlessly shoveling food in my mouth. My mantra gives me time to think about what I am doing moments before eating and focuses on my appreciation of food. I want to feel that food and I are on good terms. It does not have control over me. It complements me and my life. When we rush while eating, we become stuffed before our mind/body can register that it is satisfied. We lose that calm and happy state. The peaceful interaction with food becomes one of frustration and negativity. I despise hearing people say, "I ate too much," "Man, I am stuffed," "Ugh, I feel sick." Granted, I do this on occasion, but it is rare because the only person to blame for these negative feelings is *me*. Had I slowed down and made eating a peaceful and enjoyable experience, these feelings would never be felt. By saying I am "allowing" food inside me, it gives me a complete sense of power over food. Never the opposite. Eating should always be a pleasurable, positive, wonderful experience.

Think about your normal routine when you eat. Write it down. Think about how it currently is and what could be improved. Do you hurry through meals? Feel stressed? Anxious? Do you savor what you are consuming? Next, think about how you want to experience meals. Do you want them to be pleasurable? Happy? Calm? A positive experience? What can you do to go from the current meal experience to the one you desire?

—— **CRITICAL POINTS:** ——

- Always sit down when eating.
- If you feel rushed or hurried, take a few breaths and relax before taking your first bite.
- Say a brief premeal mantra in your head and show love and gratitude for what you are putting inside your body.
- Savor each bite of food and recognize that you are eating because you are hungry and not because you feel pressured or obligated, or any other negative emotional reason.
- Ponder about how your current or typical mealtime experience is. Think of a few words that describe this experience.
- How do you want your mealtime experience to be? Calm? Happy? Relaxing? Easy? Use a few words to describe your ideal encounter with food and eating. Think of those words as you eat to help ground you and help you feel centered.

—————

Am I Enjoying This?

Another technique that has helped me stay "binge free" is to ask myself, "Am I enjoying this?" Too often we eat things that do not taste good at all! How often do we stop ourselves and ask if we are really enjoying what we are putting in our mouths? Never. I was eating pasta the other night with my children and after taking three bites thought to myself, *This doesn't even taste good.* I don't even like lasagna or red sauce. Instantly I put my fork down and was done. How often do we put food in our mouths without thinking? Too often. Growing up, my mother used to always say, "We are not garbage disposals." We are not. Our bodies are not this "throw all the waste inside" living containers that we put trash in. Much of the food we consume should be considered trash. It does nothing as far as benefiting us, nourishing us, or giving us life and energy. Many foods do the opposite. They suck life and energy from our bodies. I can't tell you how many times I started out on a binge, but it ended quickly when I realized I absolutely hated what I was putting in my mouth. It was not enjoyable. I was doing it for the mere sake of wanting something to chew on or because of the thoughts and emotions inside me were bubbling up and I wanted to stuff them back down.

If you find yourself wanting something to put in your mouth, grab some gum, ice chips, or carbonated water to satisfy that desire to eat. Each time you eat, say your mantra, begin eating, then ask yourself after each bite if you are thoroughly enjoying what you are consuming. If you aren't, then stop! No one is holding a gun to your head. You are the only person putting food in your mouth. You have full control to stop at any time. You may write the foods you don't like (that maybe you thought you did) down if you wish. You can keep track of which foods you enjoy and don't enjoy. You can rate it, use a numeric scale, whatever you fancy. I simply want you to ask the question in your head each time you eat "Am I enjoying this?" Again, feel free to push the food away if you aren't. Throw it away. Or get up and walk away from it. No one is forcing you to eat. I never make my kids eat food they don't care for (unless it is fruit or veggies) or clean their plates. That is setting them up to overeat when they are not truly hungry and to not recognize that food is supposed to be good-tasting (in a fresh orange kind of way, not like a Snickers bar!). Our bodies are amazing and phenomenal living organisms and need to be cared for and treated as such!

—— CRITICAL POINTS: ——

- Ask yourself while eating if you are enjoying the food. If not, then put the food down and walk away.
- Realize you're in full control and have all the power when eating.

I Can Say No?

I had a client I was coaching not too long ago who had lost a considerable amount of weight. He said one of the biggest challenges he was facing was how to tell others no when they offered him food. He explained to me that he felt a horrible guilt when he turned down edible items that were offered to him. I reassured him over and over to never feel guilty for turning down food. Most of it was junk and he knew he would lose control if he ate it, so he unleashed his absolute strength and power, said no thanks and walked away. If a coworker put treats on his desk, he would quickly put them away and save them for his kids. You are under no obligation to eat for any reason. You have the right to say **no** to food any time you please. Whether it is offered by your mom, a coworker, or a waitress at a restaurant, or if you are standing naked in front of the open fridge at three in the morning craving a snack. Saying no is a beautiful and powerful tool that you need to exercise more often! I have stood in front of the pantry many times and had to yell out loud at myself, "Get out! You don't want to eat! You aren't hungry!"

—— **CRITICAL POINTS:** ——

- Exercise your power and strength by saying no
- Never feel obligated to eat, no matter who is offering it or what is being offered.

Affirmations

If I have a day where I did not have time to meditate or do any form of visualization first thing in the morning, I feel as though something is missing. I absolutely love affirmations. They can be done anytime, anywhere, and are a quick and easy way to flood your mind with positivity and peace. If I am having a rough day, I will say them dozens of times. Whether or not I believe them when I am saying them, they help me redirect my thoughts and attention to something positive that I can control. Create some of your own! Here are a few of my favorites:

"I am calm. I am at peace. I have no desire to hurt my body. I have no desire to hurt my spirit. My mind is filled with gratitude for myself and others. I am pure love. Only love fills me. I am powerful. I have more strength than I ever imagined. I eat to have energy. I do not eat my emotions. I allow myself to feel emotions and release them."

You have begun using the purge-free techniques from chapter 5 and are rocking them! Your purges are becoming more and more infrequent. You have moved on to the binge-free techniques and are beginning to gain a sense of empowerment and freedom as you start to realize how fun and easy it is to have control over food and your interactions with it. Eating is starting to feel enjoyable a little more each day as you allow a calm and relaxed energy to flood your body. Your anxiety surrounding food and eating is decreasing. Saying no to food at any time is exhilarating. Now, let's work on what is going on in that beautiful mind of yours!

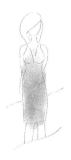

Chapter 7

STOP EATING
YOUR EMOTIONS

You Are Loved

My dear friend, no matter what challenges you face in life, the most important thing to know is that you are not alone. Growing up and even still, I feel very much in a world all by myself. I try to deal with things on my own. I push people away without trying to. While I was healing, I longed for someone to care. I wanted to show everyone around me how strong and amazing I was, that I could handle anything. For years I pushed my emotions down, down, down. Down so deep that no one, not even I, could find them. Doing that caused a lot of anxiety, depression, and frustration. No one saw the sad, lonely, depressed inner side of me. I was the nice girl who was friends with everyone, the amazing girl who was so good at putting on a show—happy, smiling—but dying on the inside.

When we push our emotions deep down inside ourselves the inner turmoil always leaks out in other ways. To deal with the inner chaos and damaged emotional state, I turned outwardly to food for comfort. As you are. I can't tell you the number of times I have thought about you. Longed to reach out and wrap my arms around you. I've cried myself to sleep so many nights wanting to talk to you. To console your aching heart. To let you know you weren't alone in this battle. Were you behind me in your car this morning as I dropped my kids off at school? Across the field at the park utterly alone in your thoughts of self-loathing? If I had listened to that nagging feeling and called you, maybe it would have stopped you from putting another Twinkie in your mouth. Had I invited you to yoga with me, maybe your food bender would not have begun during that hour of weakness; maybe the class would have given you the strength you needed to say no for one more day. Maybe a week. Maybe indefinitely. Had I let you complain to me at the office or offered to go to dinner with you and listen to your struggles, maybe you would have seen that small light of hope that you needed to not turn to another unhealthy and destructive outlet. Counting the times, I longed for a phone call, a hug or kind word from someone, anyone, would be impossible. I prayed to God that he would heal me. Maybe I am that calming miracle you need to prevent you from hitting your kids because the anger for yourself is so great that you can't contain the emotions from spilling out onto your beautiful babies. I've been there. Been in the dark abyss. I reach out to you now with love in my heart. With a desire to help heal your wounds. I know how you are feeling right now. As if there is no way out of this dark place that you have allowed yourself to sink down into. I am telling you now my dearest friend, you are on your way out. Put your belief in the potter who molded and shaped you so beautifully. Put your trust in me. I've been down that road. It took me many years to find that small light in the corner of the dark cave. I don't want it to take you years. You've hit a breaking point, or else you wouldn't be reading these words right now. It's a must. You can't continue this way of living and your desperation to change keeps you up at night. Feel that beautiful desire. Let it grow inside you. Get excited. Change is coming. A new life is coming. It's within your reach and you are going to take hold and run with it.

Burn That BS

So much of what we believe is false. If you were to stop for a moment and observe your thoughts you would recognize that most of them are negative, self-deprecating, and defeating. Very little of what plays in your mind is accurate. However, you have replayed these thoughts over and over that now they have become programmed into the hard drive of your mind and accepted as truth. A belief is simply a thought you think over and over and over. For many years I did not wear shorts because my legs were thick. Was this true? Well, I told myself my legs were thick and thick girls shouldn't show their legs. Only skinny girls with thin legs should wear shorts. Isn't that complete BS? This is one of the many false beliefs I have allowed to control me and my mind, and in turn, my actions. Stop for a moment and think about your self-talk. What is playing in your mind right now? What is playing all day every day? What are you thinking? What are you telling yourself? How about those things that you swear by? I must eat dinner at by 6:00 p.m. because eating late at night makes me store fat. I must eat breakfast every day. I need one hundred ounces of water of day. Sugar is the devil. Fat will clog your arteries. Are these truths? Or are these things we have heard, or told ourselves or been told by others, repeated over and over in our minds until they became programmed and held as beliefs.

I am not here to debate whether you should eat breakfast, stop eating by a certain time, cut or not cut out food groups, or follow the food pyramid, but the fact is, we have a lot of personal rules about ourselves (and our lives) that we live by that are complete baloney! Contemplate for a moment about what you think about yourself, your body, your health, your willpower, and your strength. Think about your determination.

About your life. What lies have others told you? What lies have you told yourself?

This next exercise is a simple one I started doing years ago that has been instrumental in helping me transform and heal myself from my incorrect thinking and actions. It takes a little bit of time to complete. Is it worth it? Every second of it. You can repeat this as many times as you wish until you feel like the lies that are stained in your mind have been bleached out. The beautiful thing is, when those lies start to infiltrate your mind again, the second they enter, you can *burn* them.

I want you to take a few minutes or more, depending on how hard it may be for you to recall past information, to think back over your life. Go back as early as you can remember and pull out of your memory bank all the unfair, incorrect, unjustified falsities that people have said about you. Or things you have repeated about yourself that you eventually took in as truth but aren't true! Anything that does not contribute to the person you want to be. For me, it was me telling myself that I could never be thin. That I would always be a bigger girl and struggle with my weight. That I would never be able to wear a two-piece swimming suit because of the embarrassment of my stretch marks on my lower abdomen.

Until two years ago, I never wore shorts because I always thought my legs were too thick. I can't tell you the times that I played over and over in my mind that I would never be able to overcome my addiction with food or have a healthy mind free from destructive thoughts. Or that I would always be a bulimic and laxative abuser because I had no self-control. For sure God would never love me because of the horrible things that I was doing to the body he had given me. I could never have a healthy relationship or marriage because of the emotional damage being sexually abused had caused me. What lies have you believed? Not only lies about your health, fitness, weight, appearance, and so on, but what about lies regarding your love life, your family life, your finances, your social life, your spirituality? What about your dreams? Your aspirations? Write these lies down as they come to you, so you don't forget. List them all. As many as you can. Mine would have looked like this:

- I have thick legs
- God doesn't love me
- I will always be a bulimic
- I will always abuse laxatives
- I can't wear a two-piece swimming suit
- Chubby girls shouldn't show their legs
- I am not loveable
- I will never have a heathy relationship/marriage
- I will never be "skinny"
- I will always be addicted to food

- I don't know how to handle my emotions in a healthy way
- I am weak
- I am not patient
- It's too hard to have self-control
- Food is my friend, my outlet
- I must have done something wrong to have been sexually abused
- I will never forgive myself
- I will never forgive those who have hurt me
- I will never love myself
- I am disgusting because only a disgusting person binges and vomits
- Nothing will cure me
- I could never write a book, no one wants to hear what I have to say

Lies! Absolute lies! I laugh as I write these old beliefs because I no longer believe any of them.

Now make your list.

Once the paper you have in front of you is filled with false beliefs (lies), I want you to hold it close to your heart. As you breathe deeper, feel all the energy inside you that has been taking up space from these lies flow into the paper and out of your body.

Next, I want you to take a match or lighter, the paper, and go somewhere safe. Obviously, let's be smart here. Hold the paper out in front of you and light it on fire. At some point you are going to have to put the paper down, so it doesn't burn you. Put it in a fire proof container or on the cement and let it continue to burn. Observe those lies that you believed for so long dissipate. Watch as all those lies go up in flames. They are no longer a part of you.

As the paper is almost completely incinerated, let go and watch the burning ashes fall to the ground, scattering quickly and effortlessly. The lies are gone. The false beliefs are gone. They no longer exist in your mind. You are freed from them. You are now free to think new thoughts and create correct and amazing beliefs.

After you have completed this exercise, feel the huge mental space that is freed up, your mind is now ready to be filled with new and amazing beliefs about yourself.

Recap:
- Take out a piece of paper
- Write down all false beliefs that you think about yourself or others think or have thought about you.
- Hold the paper close to your heart and allow the emotional energy from these false beliefs to leave your body and become soaked up into the paper.

- Take a match or lighter and set all the lies on fire, making sure to have a safe spot to put the paper as it burns.
- Watch the paper go up in flames and the ashes scatter and dissipate.
- If you do not wish to physically do this, then close your eyes and perform the burning act in your mind. It will be just as good!
- Feel the space that is freed up from releasing all the lies you have held.
- Repeat this any time you start to feel those thoughts return. All you do is close your eyes and see the beliefs burning up in flames. Easy as that!

Another good visualization I love to do is to see myself writing each false belief on a piece of paper, stuffing it into a balloon, blowing up the balloon, releasing it, and watching it float up into the sky and out of your life. As the balloon floats away, you can feel the thoughts being released from you. Use all your senses when performing these exercises.

New Me

As I mentioned in chapter 5, I used to watch a video of myself binging and purging every morning. I stopped after a few months because it was negative and made me feel depressed.

Instead, I started to visualize my *new self* every morning before I got out of bed. I no longer wanted to focus on what I was. I wanted to start seeing the new version of myself. The person I knew I could be. I keep my phone and headphones next to my bed and turn on relaxing piano music every morning. I let my mind go wild. The video that plays (I still perform this) in my head is always the same. I am running on a sandy beach. The sun is warm against my skin. I am in a beautiful white bikini. Something I had fantasized of wearing my entire life. Complete bliss. Happy beyond words. Smiling. Sun hat on. My kids running on the shore just a few feet away from me, laughing and dancing. Every morning I wake up and lay in bed for about ten minutes and perform this. If you wake up at 6:00 a.m., great. Start waking up at 5:50. I promise it won't kill you. It will be the best ten minutes of your day! I don't look at Facebook, the news, emails, or anything negative. Our minds are most impressionable first thing in the morning. I use my imagination to see the life I want to live. The New Me! It starts my day in such a way that empowers my soul. Some mornings I will visualize how my day will play out. I see myself having an awesome day at work, getting along with my boss and coworkers, saying no to the doughnuts at the office, changing the negative thoughts that pop into my head to positive ones. I want you to start fantasizing about the new you. The you that is strong, powerful, in complete control of your life, and, above all, bulimia free.

Allow Yourself to Feel

I had to catch myself the other day from telling my son to suck it up and quit whining about his schoolteacher, who, he thinks, doesn't like him. Why would we ever tell another human being not to feel a certain emotion? Why, when we were given by our amazing Creator, the ability to experience emotions, would we discourage any human from allowing themselves that right? Instead, we encourage suppression and question *why* and *what* we are feeling as though it were a bad thing. I want you to post notes around your house that say, "Feel it." While healing from bulimia, I often had to remind myself to let myself feel the emotions swarming inside me. I would walk to the couch and sit for a moment and let myself understand why I was reaching for something to put in my mouth instead of acknowledging what was going on inside me. While I sat for a moment, I would let any emotions flow through my body, then allow them to pass out of my being.

———— **CRITICAL POINTS:** ————

- Do not discount your feelings. Ever!
- Allow yourself to feel any and all emotions

- Acknowledge them, feel them, and allow your mind and body to release them
- Do not dwell on them
- Do not give them unnecessary power
- Free yourself from them
- If needed, use the burn that BS or balloon-release techniques/meditation

---

How Am I Feeling?

"How am I feeling" goes right along with allow yourself to feel. I ask myself, "How am I feeling?" frequently. Sometimes hourly. I love knowing that at any moment I can change the way I feel. If I start to feel insecure, defensive, stressed, anxious, or negative in any way, I instantly acknowledge the emotion and let it pass through me. I will repeat in my head, "Noelle, it's OK that you feel insecure right now. There is a beautiful female in front of you and you feel threatened, inadequate and insecure. You know that you are just as amazing as her. You have so many phenomenal qualities. God made you both special and unique. Send her nothing but love."

As soon as I acknowledge the emotion, I pivot, and quickly change the thought I was thinking that made me feel insecure to a positive and uplifting thought. We can't experience feelings of love and feelings of hate at the same time. If I become angry and start to have negative feelings inside me, I instantly allow my body to become flooded with love for that person. I pivot my thoughts and quickly change the thought to the opposite of what I was thinking. I will close my eyes for a moment and do the New Me exercise. My mental state and mood are instantly improved. If able, give that person a hug, hand shake, a kind word, or a kind gesture. Don't be consumed with hate or any negative emotion. Life is short. Don't waste your precious time and energy on negative emotions.

Being sexually abused as a child left me with a lot of hatred inside. Resentment. Absolute hostility. Obviously, that did me no good. I had to let go of those negative feelings. I had to send love to the person who hurt me. I had to thank him in my heart that he gave me the opportunity to overcome those feelings, to overcome bulimia, to recognize my absolute strength. I let those feelings go. They no longer plague or torment me. The memories do not haunt me. Ever. They are gone. Where there were once horrific dreams and memories, now there is only love, peace, kindness, happiness, and hope. Do the same with your negative feelings for any person who has hurt you. Whether you were abused, as I was, or if someone hurt you mentally or emotionally, let those bottled up feelings go. Send them nothing but love.

If you have hurt another person, you must forgive yourself and allow healing to take place. I have hurt others. I have made mistakes. I could sit and wallow in my pity and guilt but there is no longer room for that in my life. I sent love and forgiveness to myself and let it all go. I know you can do the same. You are beautiful and amazing. I tell my sweet children that yesterday is in the past and today is a new day. A chance to be better. A chance to start fresh. Take time each day to perform affirmations that build and uplift you. Focus on what things you love and appreciate about yourself. You are reading these words right now, so I know for a fact that you are an advocate for your well-being, you love yourself enough to improve your mind, you love to learn, and you are striving to be better. There you go, four amazing things you can show gratitude for and that you can repeat all day every day to build yourself up!

Instead of shutting your emotions up inside you, causing all sorts of inner turmoil and outer ailments, acknowledge what you are feeling at any given moment and let the feelings flow through you. Realize that we were given emotions for a reason. Don't discredit them. Don't suppress them. Don't burry them. Feel them. Give thanks and gratitude for your emotions and that they are a wonderful and beautiful thing! You don't have to use food, alcohol, drugs, or any negative act or substance to numb yourself any longer. You do not have to be afraid of feeling, as I once was. Face those emotions head on. Write down what you are feeling. Talk to someone. Eating your emotions only hurts you.

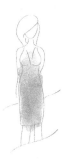

Chapter 8

How could God allow this problem into my life? Why would God give me something as difficult as this? Why would God allow my life to be destroyed by my thoughts and my actions? Why would God allow another human to hurt me? Doesn't God love me? Questions like this have gone through my mind and are currently going through yours. Would I be lying if I said I had a definite answer for you? Yes. I can only say a few things to satisfy your questioning mind. To calm you.

First, the Creator of this universe loves you. My words cannot express the magnitude of love that always surrounds you. Always. You are special and unique. You were no accident. You have meaning and significance.

Second, my dear friend, there is beauty in contrast. If we do not go through challenges in life, we will never grow and expand. Let's suppose you go to the gym every morning and desperately want definition and muscle tone on your body. However, if you don't take the dumbbells up from five to ten pounds, you will never grow that small bicep muscle that is longing to enlarge. We are no different. We must be molded, shaped, and stretched if we want to grow. Emotionally. Physically. Mentally. In the thick of being molded, it does not feel good. If I am being honest here, I would have to say it feels downright torturous. Painful. But there is so much beauty in your challenges. The satisfaction when coming out on the other side is monumental. I did not feel this way a few years ago. I did not see my battle with bulimia and self-loathing as a positive thing and would have fought anyone who told me otherwise. Looking back, I know the dark abyss I was trapped in was transforming me. I wouldn't take back any of my experiences. I love every second that I live my new life. It makes me grateful for where I have been.

Third, you will always get what you look for in life. The Source has given each of us the ability to see good and bad, right and wrong, beauty and ugliness, light and dark. When we focus intensely on one end of the spectrum it is impossible to see the opposite. If I constantly look for reasons to be sad and hateful, then I will continue to find more reasons. More than I can handle. There will be an endless supply of negative thoughts and experiences around every corner. This was how

I lived for years. I could only see the bad. The ugly. The damage. I lived in a "pity me" state of mind. It was when I stopped looking for the bad that I stopped seeing it. I was sexually abused; lots of people are. I was raised in a big family and felt overlooked at times, so what! I got divorced and had three little children I was supporting on my own, wooptie-freakin'-do. I struggled with an eating disorder for twenty years—cry me a river! Other people are more successful, more beautiful, more amazing than me in a lot of ways—and your point is? I can sit in a corner and pout all day long and feel sorry for myself and my existence, but what would that accomplish? I can blame the God above, my parents, my boss, my emotions, the neighbor next door, or a nonempathetic therapist for all the wrong things that have happened to me, but in all reality, none of that matters any more. None of it!

——— CRITICAL POINTS: ———

- You are loved! Start feeling that love.
- There is beauty in contrast. Instead of hating the bad, start loving it and showing gratitude for it. It is making you more amazing and stronger every day!
- Look for the good in all things. The road you're driving on, the cat in the yard, the food you eat, the job you have.

- The more you look for the amazing things in life, the more you will find them!
- The same goes for the negative. If you look for the bad, the ugly, and all the injustices of the world, you will without a doubt find them. Don't waste your precious time and energy on the bad.

As a registered nurse, I understand the intricate workings of the human body. It's mind-blowing to say the least. There is no way that anything less than a supernatural creator was the architect of these bodies, including the mind. You may disagree that there is a God above and that is totally OK; however, you cannot disagree with the absolute complexity of each of us, or with this universe! Some things are simply out of our control and more than we can physically or mentally handle on our own. I was raised in a religious family but have not been religious for several years. However, I am still very spiritual. Very in tune to the divinity of all things and the intuitive feelings each of us possesses. I believe strongly in synchronicity, or meaningful coincidences. I believe things happen for a reason, that our thoughts create our lives and what we call reality. I know without a doubt that deep down in our beings, each of us is good and pure. Things happen for a reason. You are reading these words right now, and that to me is a sign that you needed to find my words and feel my love and desire for you to be healed.

The night I drove up the mountain to my home after my last massive (and I mean massive) binge, was a night that I will never forget. I prayed that night that God would cause me to drive off the cliff. My life was not worth living any longer. I was so exhausted. Tired of being controlled by my emotions, food, and life's circumstances. I wanted so desperately to die. God had another plan in mind. There was something that I had not accomplished. A divine purpose I had not yet fulfilled. In the midst of the darkness and chaos you are feeling at this moment, you might not recognize the divine purpose in front of you, but there is a plan. Your plan. There is peace. You must stop for a moment and recognize what it is. "I have no idea what my purpose is Noelle. There is not a divine plan for me." Bull! Stop that negative thinking right now. You are absolute perfection. To find that plan you need to give your bulimia to God, uncover your divine path, feel closer to a higher power, and put it to the test.

Give It to God

You can continue to be eaten alive by the mistakes you have made or the absolute injustices that others have done to you. You can wake up every morning and replay these terrible scenes in your head, let the emotions that surround the act consume you, and live day in and day out in a state of pity, despair, anger, or hatred. Or you can simply let it go. Let it all go. Turn all the anguish that is inside you right now over to God. I like to imagine my feelings as a huge boulder that I carry on my back between my shoulder blades (this is where I carry my stress). When I start to feel a heaviness weighing me down, I visualize myself handing that boulder over to the universe, God, the Source, whatever you label it.

Whether you are fifteen, forty-five, or ninety-two, you can give the unwanted feelings inside you away. You no longer have to keep them. There is a force greater than any of us, greater than this universe. You have burned those BS thoughts that have plagued you, released all the negative and destructive memories, allowed them to effortlessly float out of your mind and your life, and replaced them with who and what you now want to be. Do not allow anything that does not build you up to take up space in your mind. Remember, one of the reasons conventional therapy might not have worked for you, is because you hashed and rehashed the horrible experiences and thoughts until they had so much power that the momentum you allowed them to gain kept on going. Stop the momentum. Do not give those experiences any more power. Downplay them? Yes, downplay them. Minimize them. Stop talking about them. Let them go. Give them to God.

Test It

Are you someone who needs proof? Needs something tangible? I am. I stood in the shower many years ago alone with my thoughts. Thoughts about being abused as a young child flooded my mind. They overwhelmed me. Sickened me. I knelt in the shower that day and prayed to my Creator that he would take it all away. I put it to the test. I told God (or whatever you want to call this power) that if he would remove this hurt inside me, that I would do my best to live in a way that would make him proud. I promised to be the best person I could be. Promised I would love my children the way they needed to be loved. I would find others like me and help them on their journey to healing. Am I better now? Was I good on my promise? Most days I am. Am I perfect? No. Far from it. I swear, drink coffee, have an occasional alcoholic beverage, yell at my kids, and experience occasional road rage. Does this make me bad? No. I am a work in progress, and I forgive myself for the weakness I have. I am forgiving of myself and others. But I put God to the test. In his time, he helped me. Healed me. Allowed me to move past the demon that I couldn't conquer on my own. I handed off my bulimia boulder that weighted me down for too long, to God. I keep myself in a state that allows me to feel intuition. To feel God working magic in my life.

We all have a guidance system inside us. We were not thrown down onto this planet without an innate way to navigate through living. We all feel. Good or bad, right or wrong. We have our emotions. Let them guide you. If something brings peace and a feeling of calm and joy inside you, then obviously that is an indicator that you are on the right path. If something brings negative feelings or inner turmoil, then it is an indicator that you are not doing the correct thing. You might think you are past the point of feeling. Maybe you see yourself as unworthy or not a "good" person. That is the biggest bunch of crap I've ever heard. No one is ever past the point of being good or feeling positive feelings. That is what you are telling yourself and those lies must stop. I have not met you. I do not know you. But I can sense your goodness. Your beauty. Your amazing inner strength. There is power that radiates through this universe that beams down on you at any given moment. Use your emotions and the power of the universe to guide you through healing yourself of this eating disorder.

Finding Your Divine Purpose

What brings you absolute happiness? What brings you peace? What makes you feel as though your life is worth living? Whatever it is, do more of it. Live from that state of peace and happiness as often as you can. When I think about helping others, it makes me light up inside. When I think about being an amazing mom, I become giddy. When I hear someone say I helped them in some way, changed their life, helped them recognize something they didn't see before, I feel a warmth spread over my body and I know that is my purpose. What is yours? Write them down. What do you love? What makes you happy? What gives you peace?

How to Feel Closer to a Higher Power

When you have denied the existence of a creator or stood in a place in your life where you are unable to feel the presence of one, it's hard to allow your mind to go there. I was raised in a religious home, but that does not mean that I had a true knowledge of God. I followed what everyone else was doing, road along on their coattails and pretended as though I was a devout Christian. It was not until I hit rock bottom and had that undying desire to know I was not alone, that I found God. For years I pleaded, "God, where art thou? Please, Lord, do not let this continue any longer. God, please help me out of this dark place." I would promise the Lord that if he would help me, I would change my life. I would be more like him. That does not mean I go around preaching religion, or attend church every Sunday, or quote Bible verses; it means I strive to be more like God in word and action: kind, loving, understanding, slower to anger, enjoying life, laughing.

For years these pleadings became stronger; then I realized why I had not been receiving any direction or guidance. My life was complete chaos. It was constant chatter. Work. Kids. Noise. I had to put myself in a place where I could hear and feel intuitive guidance. That's when I realized the things I needed to do: meditation, yoga, lying on my bed and relaxing, positive affirmations. Once I quieted my mind, I started to feel something. Call it God, a Holy Spirit, my inner being. I started to sense that there was something, someone, a powerful energy and magnificent sense of well-being surrounding me always. I stopped feeling utterly alone. I had this amazing epiphany that I no longer needed food as a friend, a companion. I no longer had a desire to punish myself. I started having this knowing inside me that I was special. I had a purpose. I began to feel an overwhelming love for myself. This love was so strong that I began to think, I love myself too much to hurt myself. What things can you do to put yourself into a place that allows this sense of well-being?

- Meditation
- Yoga
- Music
- Fasting
  - o There is nothing more wonderful than weakening the carnal body to feel more receptive to feelings/

intuition. I fast for twenty-four hours every week
to strengthen my mental and emotional power

- Writing, verbalizing, or thinking things you are
  grateful for
- Affirmations
  - o Our words have amazing power and strength.
    I begin every day with a few simple positive
    affirmations about myself.
  - o I love my beautiful and perfect body
  - o I am powerful and strong beyond imagining
  - o I am victorious and can conquer any challenge
    that comes before me
  - o Peace radiates through me on this new day like
    a wave washes over the sand and clears away any
    blemishes
  - o My life is perfect. At this moment, I am exactly
    where I am supposed to be.
  - o I look forward to each day because it brings with
    it a new me

The list above are some wonderful examples. Can you think
of a few more things that you like to do to bring you closer to
God, make you feel more grounded and peaceful, or help you
become more intuitive? Also, create your own affirmations that
resonate with you and post them all around your house.

God, where art thou? He is right beside you, friend. Constant. Strong. Ready to take the heavy boulder you are holding and give you freedom. To break the chains. To free you from bondage. To help you feel loved. To allow you to forgive yourself. To guide you as you strengthen your relationship with yourself and stop the binges and purges. To help you change your thoughts. To make you recognize that you are loved. He is there. Put yourself in a place where you can feel the Creator's love for you. Do those things that you enjoy and bring satisfaction. Find your purpose. Be glad for this journey you have traveled. Recognize that the potter has been molding and shaping you. Stretching you to greatness. The contrast has been challenging, but now you are on your way to being free. Free from bulimia. Free from addiction. Free from negative thoughts and behaviors. You are finally free to live. There will be moments of weakness. Times that you may relapse. But they will become few and far between.

You have mastered the purge and binge techniques. You have changed your thinking and begun loving and forgiving yourself. You are discovering that forgiving others is easy. Thoughts of love and gratitude swarm your mind. You have reached out to God for additional help. Given the fight to him and found peace. You have thought of ways you can allow intuition into your life, which in turn will help guide you to your path and purpose in life. You are making amazing strides! Bulimics also find other ways to torture and control their lives once the bulimic cycle has ceased. We must stop punishing ourselves with other means, whether a binge has occurred or not. The two most commonly used modes are laxatives and exercise. These can become as addictive and dangerous as binging and purging.

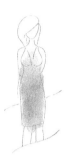

Chapter 9
STOP PUNISHING YOURSELF

As much as a bulimic wants control, they are very much out of control, not just with their thoughts and eating patterns, but with ways to maintain their weight. Once the purges ended and the binges became less and less frequent, I still struggled with laxative and exercise abuse as a form of punishment.

Laxatives

It was a beautiful morning when I knocked on the front door of the home of my first patient. An admit. Forty-five to sixty minutes max, or so I thought. The wife let me in and pointed up the stairs to where her husband was. As I slowly made my way toward the far room at the end of the hall, I felt it, that light cramping and gnarly feeling in my bowels that began about ten to twelve hours after taking a laxative. I began to panic. I had twenty minutes. Thirty tops. I rushed through vitals and assessment and quickly looked at the incision site. The cramping became stronger. My bowels were churning nicely. The egg salad sandwich, potato chips, three cookies, and a milkshake mini binge were mixing in a nice bath of bile juices just as I wanted. Ready to make their exit quickly. It was never pretty.

Talk about horrible timing. I took the laxatives fourteen hours ago thinking I would have plenty of time to do my thing before work. Wrong. I began to sweat profusely under my scrubs. I felt drops of perspiration run down my back and in between my breasts. How long could I squeeze my glutes together and hold it in? Ten minutes maybe. The cramping grew persistently strong. Why did I take fourteen of them? My usual dose was six, but lately the little orange pills have been taking longer to work so I made sure they would kick in within ten hours by doubling the dose. Again, not smart. I closed out my visit, walked back down the stairs and hurriedly said goodbye to the wife as I closed the front door behind me. I paused for a second midway to the car and prayed. I was dripping sweat and clenching my behind together so tight I could have held a penny in a firm grip. I got into my car and clenched the steering wheel. My entire body tensed as the cramping in my bowels became uncontrollable. I can do this. I can do this. All I had to do was make it down the hill to the gas station bathroom. As

I pulled out of the driveway it hit like a tsunami. The release felt amazing, but the warm liquid sickened me as it ran down my legs and puddled underneath me on the leather seat. My scrubs absorbed what they could, but the rest just flowed off onto the beautiful floor of my Lexus. I pulled off onto a side street and down into a deserted construction area. Praise the lord. No one in sight. I jumped out of the car, grabbed the blue chuck pad I kept for wound care visits, and the packet of disposable washcloths and began peeling my clothes off. I left the scrubs, panties, dirty pad and soiled washcloths on the side of the dirt road. Back in the car I noticed I had missed some. Again, I wiped my legs off. I could see chunks of egg in my stool. *How could I be so unbelievably disgusting?* I thought over and over. I drove home, jumped in the shower, and cleaned my car as best I could before another massive eruption occurred. Another wonderful crapping experience. This is the sad and cruel reality of laxative abuse. Another way to punish myself after a small binge.

Is this you? Are you a laxative abuser? How about a compulsive exerciser? Do you starve yourself for days on end after a massive binge and/or purge? Do you feel as though you must punish yourself after eating a little more than you wanted? Do you feel as if you just performed a hideous crime by eating "forbidden" foods and now must torture yourself by pooping, burning off excess calories, or starving yourself back to normal?

This self-inflicted aftermath is just as damaging mentally and physically for the body. Not to mention downright nasty.

Twenty-plus years of being a bulimic made my bowels almost nonfunctional. If I do not take three laxatives once a week, I cannot poop. At all. It is a miserable feeling being full of crap. Inability to have normal bowel movements is a horrible side effect of bulimia. But because I would consider myself very obsessive and/or compulsive at times, I must be cautious not to abuse the laxatives. As you can read from my account above, I abused them heavily for a few years before realizing that the side effects were getting worse and worse. Initially the side effects were only bloating, cramping, and nausea. Then it turned into severe nausea, itching of my skin, severe muscle aches, weakness, and light-headedness. They also made me hungrier and worsened my food cravings, not to mention the absolute embarrassment of having explosive diarrhea, frequent accidents, and throwing a lot of cute clothes away!

As you begin to have less frequent binges, the need for laxatives will decrease. Taking laxatives after a binge helps a bulimic rid themselves of extra food and brings a sense of feeling thin. It was not easy to stop abusing the orange miracle pills, but as my mind-set changed and the desire to have complete control over my thoughts and actions grew, I knew any excessive behavior had to go! If you struggle with laxative abuse, be diligent in using the binge-free techniques to keep yourself in control of food and avoidance of being overly stuffed. If your bowels are slow, use natural means first. Increase water intake to soften stool, keep your body hydrated and satisfied, increase your fiber, and stay active. If these do not work, take the recommended number of laxatives. I try to take them only once a week so as to not allow my body to become overly dependent on them.

As a personal trainer, health coach, registered nurse, and very active mom, I understand the importance and benefits of regular exercise on our health. However, I know of many men and women who spend hours at the gym. This is silly! I knew a woman who would bring her food wrappers and set them on the treadmill console, so she knew how many calories she had to burn off. Let's go back to our thinking for a moment. There's got to be a balance on all things in our lives. If we are spending three hours at the gym to burn off calories from a binge or live in constant fear of "getting fat," we are neglecting the most important things in our lives: our families. Bulimia has stolen hours from my life already. There is no way that obsessive exercising is going to sneak its way into my life. Exercise is meant to be fun and enjoyable. Not torture. Not punishment. Remember that the more we exercise, the more our body craves calories to replace those that were lost. You are causing your body to want to binge on food when you exercise in an extended compulsive manner, not the opposite. Some exercise is beneficial, but when a body is not getting proper nutrition and is being pushed to the point of danger, injury can result. Stress fractures decreased sex drive, hormonal imbalances, tendonitis, changes in the immune system, and depression or anxiety can all ensue.

When you begin to become more intuitive with your emotions you will recognize the desire to exercise compulsively dissipates. There are days when my body is tired and the last thing I want to do is exercise. So, I don't. I do not beat myself up over it. If I feel like sleeping in or taking a nap, I do. Instead of obsessively pounding away at the gym, I take my kids for a bike ride, chase them around the park, or play hide and go seek in the house. I remind myself of my *why* when I begin to lose sight. My kids need a happy and healthy mom who isn't killing herself with food, barfing, exercise, or medicine. When my focus starts to become blurred, I take it back to the basics and remember who I was fighting this battle for. It wasn't to be a size two. To show everyone how perfect I "appear" to be. It was for my children, my happiness, and for you.

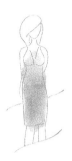

J ust as our bodies go through cycles, so do our lives. There will be times when you are on fire. When you feel amazing and invincible. As though you can conquer the world (which you can!). On the other hand, there will be times when you hit a wall, feel unusually low, or even relapse into destructive habits. That is when you stop and reevaluate what you are doing, what your *why* is, grab hold of the new you, and head that direction. You are never too far gone to come back to health, to happiness, to loving and living the life you always envisioned. I have days where I don't eat well or think well, don't act kind or patient, feel horribly alone, or want to sit in a corner and cry. The difference is that now I do not let myself stay there for very long. I do not dwell on my problems. I do not mull my emotions over and over. I accept that this is a bump in the road. I let myself feel the emotions associated with this minor bump and let them go. I forgive myself. I forgive others. I pray to God. And I look for all the things in my life that are going perfect.

I have never been addicted to drugs, tobacco, or alcohol, so I cannot speak about those addictions with certainty, but I can say for certain that until a few years ago I would have considered myself one of the worst food addicts you can imagine. I did a lot of mental and physical damage to my body. The most important part of my recovery and ability to remain bulimia free, is loving and forgiving myself. I love myself too much to have an eating disorder any longer. I love myself too much to lose control when eating. I love myself (and my little stinkers) too much to be a crappy, uninvolved mom. I forgive myself on those days when I mess up. I forgive myself for hurting others. I forgive myself for hurting my mind and body for all those years.

If you have too many obligations in your life that is causing a severe amount of stress, get rid of things. I had to cut back on the hours I was practicing nursing because of my bulimia. No one knew that was the reason, they just figured I was overly stressed. But that was the reason. I couldn't handle the stress of two nursing jobs, being a mom, health coaching, and having a suffocating eating disorder. It was too much. Bulimia will rear its ugly head when things get too stressful. Prevent that by removing things in your life that are not critical or can wait.

Learn to be OK with saying no. Put your family and yourself first. No one will fault you. I have always been a people pleaser. Saying yes to way too many things so that I wouldn't upset anyone. I'm selfish now. I am OK with saying no on a regular basis. Or I will say I have to think about it. Do not risk your health and happiness in the name of pleasing another. In the long run it only hurts you.

When I start to become overly stressed, I go back to the ways that bring me closer to God. I strive to be more intuitive and let my feelings guide me. There are days I practice yoga twice. Or meditate three times. Is this a waste of my time? Absolutely not! These ways of being closer to the universe are my saving grace. It is me being selfish and looking out for my well-being. It's me calming myself down to be a better employee, friend, lover, or mom. Next time you get overwhelmed, what are five to ten things that would relax and calm you: Meditate. Yoga. Walk. Read a book. Take a bath. Listen to calming music. Go for a drive in the country. Play with a loved pet. Do something fun with your kids (we love games). Take a nap

Make a list of how you like to relax and destress.

To remain bulimia free, we must learn to handle life's constant stresses and deal with stress in healthy ways. Take note, how are you feeling right now? Are you excited? Refreshed? Do you sense that excitement that you are on your way to being free at last?

Forgiveness

There are too many people who define themselves by their limitations. They go around seeking approval from the world and wanting everyone to feel sorry for the challenges they have gone through. I spent the first few years of my nursing career working at a women's prison. It was an eye-opening experience, to say the least. One repetitive story that many of the women told was the rehashing of the injustices that others had *done to them*. They were in prison not because of their own poor choices but because of another person's. It is easy for us to point fingers all day long. To turn any responsibility for how our lives turn out over to another and sit back and play the victim card. This story of injustice gets us nowhere. Well, it does go somewhere, but it's not a positive place. To heal from any problem, we must take ownership of what we do and how we respond to situations. As I tell my children often, we cannot change others, we can only change ourselves and how we respond. It can be as pleasant or as destructive as we make it. Earlier on I talked about taking ownership of my eating disorder and to heal I had to make it mine. Own it, and in owning it, know that I could change it.

A huge part of my healing from bulimia was forgiving those who had done me wrong. I was sexually abused as a little girl and the emotional trauma I experienced left me feeling out of control in every way. To feel in control, I used food to feel numb briefly and ultimately punish myself. I had to let go of my past so that I could move forward. As I said before, it took me a long time to hit this point. Allowing myself to turn the anguish over to God freed up emotional space that I was able to fill with the beautiful things of life. In the process of forgiving others, we must put ourselves in their situation. We focus on our problems and feelings but often overlook what they experienced. As difficult as it was, I had to get past myself and look at the person who abused me. I had to put myself in this boy's shoes. He was molested as a little boy. I had to remind myself that an injustice was done to him. That he, too, had suffered. Instead of feeling sorry for myself, I let forgiveness take over my body that day in the shower five years ago and promised I would not hate him for what he had done. I understood what he went through and my heart opened with an infinite amount of love and understanding. I no longer hated him. I no longer had thoughts of torturing and punishing him. I allowed the Creator of this world who knows all the anguish I had felt for so many years to remove the boulder from my shoulders. His strength is greater than mine. His back can withstand an infinite amount of weight. The chains of hate that bound me fell free, and I forgave my abuser completely.

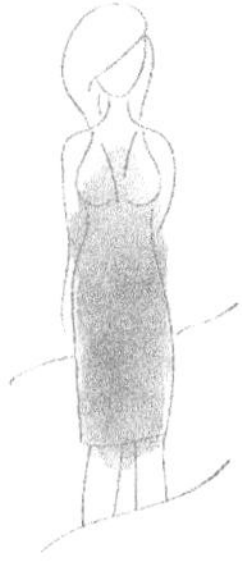

Chapter 11
FREE AT LAST

Remember back to the dark cave: trapped, bound, completely alone, crying out for help in desperation and hopelessness, wondering if you would ever escape the thick darkness that surrounded you, the feelings of despair. You never have to feel that way again my friend. You're not trapped, no longer in bondage. The suffocating feeling and mental worry of the bulimia beast is just about gone. You are free. Say that word out loud right now: free. You are free! Take a permanent marker and write boldly on a notecard, "I am free." When I finally awoke one morning and realized that I was no longer a bulimic, I cried. Those feelings flood me right now as I write this to you and tears of joy spread down my face for myself and for your amazing transformation. Destructive thoughts no longer permeate my mind. Preoccupation about food and self-punishment have scattered like ashes. The overwhelming desire to binge is a thing of the past. The desire to purge is a long-lost friend who will never come to visit again. I refuse to be controlled by her any longer. I made a list that morning, a list of all the things I wanted to do that I had not had time for because of the insane amount of time bulimia stole from me. They were things I didn't feel worthy of. I want you to sit down right now and make a list of all the things you want to do. They can be anything you wish! My list looked like this:

- Take my kids to the park and play with them (yes, play)
- Swing on the swings with my children instead of sitting in the car or on the grass and watching
- Watch an entire movie and share a bowl of popcorn with my kids
- Help my girls make cookies (I wouldn't do this, ever, for fear of starting a binge bender)
- Go to a restaurant that serves bread and have a roll before my meal and not fear losing control
- Wear a white bikini to the beach
- Buy myself a new outfit and feel beautiful in it
- Take up skiing (I've done this!)
- Take my kids ice skating (I've done this too!)

- Go to a class at the gym and not feel insecure or inadequate
- Talk about my past without any reservations
- Openly tell people (if asked of course) that I am a recovered bulimic
- Always have kind and forgiving chatter playing in my mind
- Speak kindly about myself
- Reward myself with things other than food
- Enjoy eating!
- Feel in control at parties, social gatherings, on dates, etc.
- Always feel my emotions and not burry them
- Refuse to hate or hold angry feelings toward anyone, no matter what they do or have done to me
- Accept who I am and where I've been but know that the old Noelle is long gone, never to return
- Start living a life I love and enjoy my children in complete freedom

Now make your list.

Fear of food

I used to tell myself I hated food. I would throw food away for no reason. I would throw food out my car window on a regular basis in a desperate attempt to end a binge. I loathed eating because I had no control over myself. I punished myself with food. After learning to change my thoughts about myself, my emotions, and my interaction with food, I no longer think this way. I no longer need to prove anything. I don't have to. I eat only when I am hungry. I am aware of my emotions before, during, and after eating anything. I don't have to eat my emotions. I slow down and enjoy meals. I say my premeal mantra and eat slowly, always asking how I am feeling, if the food I am eating tastes good, and I know food is now my friend. I have complete control over it. No one forces me to interact in a negative way with food but myself.

Love Thyself

I love myself more now than I ever have. I have come to an amazing place where I feel at peace with everything. I don't get worked up if things don't work out my way. In the past, so many things would piss me off, and I would bury the feelings and use food to numb, suppress, or change my emotions. Now I address the feeling, or I simply don't let it bother me. I will say in my head, "It's not worth my time getting worked up over nothing." I tell my children regularly, the only person you can control is yourself. Do not give another person or object power over you. Keep your power. Don't let another control how you feel. I am telling you this too.

Mirror, Mirror in My Hand

An amazing exercise I love to do every morning with myself and my children is to hold a small silver-framed hand mirror in front of us and repeat at least three positive aspects or qualities about ourselves. If my children say it but are not looking directly in the mirror, I make their sweet little selves repeat it! They must look directly into the mirror and into their own eyes and repeat these things. There is something magical and slightly mystical when you look directly into your own eyes and say these positive things. It reaches the soul. It's awesome to use multiple senses. "Mirror, mirror in my hand, tell me the reasons I am so grand…?" I encourage my children to perform this exercise every time they see a mirror. No matter where they are. They can say this in their head.

State three things (out loud or in your head) that you love about yourself, that make you grand!

When your mind starts to play those lies and false beliefs, pull out these three amazing qualities about yourself that you love and repeat them over and over.

Love Others

I was having a rough day. I took my kids through the McDonalds drive through to get a root beer. The lady in the next lane ordering food smiled at me and let me go ahead of her to the window to pay. She smiled at me. it was just what I needed.

She changed my day. As I pulled up to pay, I asked the girl if she would put the tab of the car behind me on mine. I pulled to the next window to get my food and looked in my rearview window. I watched as the lady behind me pulled up and the girl told her I had paid for her order. She laughed and smiled.

We lose sight of what matters most in life when we are living with a disease, addiction, or a problem that consumes us. When I was healing from bulimia, I made every effort to do more things for others. Even if it was something as simple as a smile or a compliment. It took the focus off myself and made me realize there are others in this world who are suffering just as I am. I can be the light they need just as they can help me along my journey. It's just as important to love others as it is to love yourself. Find ways that you can bring happiness to others. When you are having a rough day and begin to feel sorry for yourself or dwell on what isn't going right, perform a few small acts of kindness for another. You will be amazed at how it redirects your mind and brings about an overwhelming sense of love and happiness for yourself and others.

Just as you have, I spent so many years dying inside. Dying mentally. Dying physically. Destroying my body. Thinking perpetually negative and destructive thoughts about myself, about what I couldn't fix, about my lack, about the scarcity in my life. I loathed myself for things that were out of my control. I punished myself. Now that those thoughts and actions are gone, my life is truly in a state of bliss and freedom. I have an insane amount of mental space that I devote to the amazing person I am now. Mental space that is filled with the dreams I get to bring into reality with my children. I dwell on the love and light I can give to other people who need to recognize their amazingness and strength but can't on their own. For years I didn't love myself. I couldn't have. No one who loves themselves would use a coping mechanism like bulimia to deal with life. The thoughts of who I was rarely come into my mind. When they do, I replace them with kindness and forgiveness. I love myself. The thought of going back to that old person, to those destructive ways, is not an option. There isn't even a desire. Not physically. Not mentally.

From the second I decided to change my life and heal completely, I was never a bulimic. In my mind, I was always a recovered bulimic who no longer struggled with binges, purges, poor thinking, and so on. I was complete. Whole. Perfect. Flawless. It was an unbelievably freeing way to think. So empowering and beautiful in its entirety.

You, too, will recognize this bliss. You are already beginning to. You will come to know that the person you were always meant to be is right there below the surface. They are phenomenal. Amazing in every way. You have so much to offer the world!

One thing you must do for me is stop sabotaging your success. Stop thinking you are weak. Stop believing you are unable. Stop telling yourself this is hard. Beating bulimia is easy! You have no idea how much power you have. How great you are! If anything, you should fear your greatness. Once this beast is gone from your life, you will be able to do anything you can imagine. Nothing will seem difficult.

Be selfish. I had to come to the realization that being selfish was a good thing. We overlook our happiness and well-being for the sake of everyone and everything else. I had to say no, I am putting myself first so that I can be a better mom, a better employee, a better friend, a better lover. Do not let anyone tell you that being selfish is bad because your health and happiness is critical. Being selfish for a few years benefited my life in ways that I never imagined. I am a kinder, happier, more loving mom than I ever imagined.

Thank you, reader, for taking my hand. Thank you for embarking on this journey with me and allowing me to show you the path took to overcome bulimia. I pray with all the energy inside me that you will love yourself enough to never give up. That you now know that you are never alone in your struggle. Step out from the darkness into the light. Start living. You've got this my friend. You are amazing beyond words. That actor/actress who has starred in your movie up to this point has done it all wrong. Their mistakes have been recognized. A new star takes their place. You. It's time to take on a new role. A new you. A healed you.

ACKNOWLEDGMENTS

I suffered in silence for many years, relying little on anyone for fear of what they would think or say. How horrified would they be if they were to see the monster that I lived with? My fear of the labels or being shunned kept me in a state of silence. Living within my head with the negative tormenting thoughts was torture until I awoke to the sense that I was not alone, nor would I ever be, on this journey out of the darkness. My belief and love for what some call God, the Creator, the Source, a Heavenly Being, Elohim, Jehovah, whatever name we give, is unfathomable. I was never left alone. I never suffered in silence. My pleas for mercy were never in vain nor fell on deaf ears. Despite what I believed during my many years of anguish, the Creator was there. He pulled me from the darkness. He loosened the binds that I thought would never come free. He gave me freedom, hope, and ultimately an opportunity to bless others. Most importantly, he gave me the chance to recognize my strength and power. He made me a conqueror. I would not take back one moment of self-loathing, one second of hatred, one negative thought, one binge, one purge, one time of messing myself, one outburst of anger, or one night of wishing I would be put out of my misery. It all led me to this point in my life. To you, my dear reader.

The team at The Author Incubator has also asked me to acknowledge the Morgan James Publishing Team: David Hancock, CEO & Founder; my Author Relations Manager, Margo Toulouse; and special thanks to Jim Howard, Bethany Marshall, and Nickcole Watkins.

THANK YOU

My dear reader, I want to thank you for taking this brief journey with me. I pray this information has been as valuable for you as it was for me. However, this journey does not have to end here. Are you ready to heal your bulimia? Are you ready to experience the beautiful freedom you've been dreaming of? Are you ready to focus the time bulimia has stolen from you on more critical parts of your life? Do not waste any more time on the beast. I would be honored to work one on one with you. Please contact me at battlethebulimiabeast.com to set up a free consultation with you or a loved one. What would normally cost hundreds of dollars can be yours for free by reaching out and setting up a free consultation today!

ABOUT THE AUTHOR

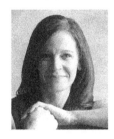

Born and raised in Galt, California, Noelle went off to Idaho to attend nursing school in 2003. She received her bachelor's in nursing in 2008 from Idaho State University and went on to practice correctional nursing and eventually home health nursing for the next ten years. Noelle is a beam of light and energy who radiates positivity wherever she goes and touches every patient's life for the better. No one would have ever known she had lived with and banished an unquenchable monster inside her.

After her divorce in 2013, Noelle's life spiraled out of control and her battle with bulimia that began as a young child reared its ugly head and took control of her life. Raising three very young children alone left her exhausted and defeated, until one night she returned home to three distraught children who needed a mom, a rock. A desperate need for change ensued.

Noelle's zest for health both mentally and physically led her to become a certified personal trainer and health coach so that she could inspire others along their journeys to complete wellness. The encounters she has had with clients encouraged her to continue giving her all with battling a long-term eating disorder. Deep in her heart, Noelle knew that there were many others struggling with the bulimic beast who needed to hear her words of encouragement and inspiration. No one should have to fight an eating disorder for twenty years before experiencing freedom.

Noelle is eager and excited to share her triumphant story and methods with those who are ready to hear them. She knows that her love for others and her desire for living a life free from the bondage of bulimia will permeate all who encounter this book. She looks forward to hearing the victorious stories of others who embark on the incredible journey of healing their minds and bodies and living the life they always dreamed.

CPSIA information can be obtained
at www.ICGtesting.com
Printed in the USA
BVHW030844280420
578706BV00001B/40